PRAISE FOR *FIT 'n*

"Lillian Easterly-Smith and Mike Smith are experts in how to really cut through and find out about how to achieve 'true health.' This impressive book is the result of years of study, training and wisdom they've learned. I highly recommend it." **– Dr. Cynthia Shaft-Toll, DC; Founder & Executive Director of Wdc Women Chiropractors**

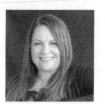

"As someone who has studied and been involved with personal fitness as well as being a person of faith, I was totally absorbed reading *Fit 'n' Faith*. Mike and Lillian Smith have captured what it means to live a healthy lifestyle from a Christian perspective. You'll read not only the **why's** but also be able to follow a step by step plan to enhance your life Physically and Spiritually. A MUST read." **– Marc Major Speaker/Coach/Personal Trainer/Radio Personality Executive Director with the John Maxwell Leadership Development Team**

"In 2010, I had an 'aha' moment. I was obese. Over 450 pounds. My blood pressure was 190/110, causing me to be on three different types of medicine. My waist measured 70" around. I needed to make some drastic changes in my life...I wanted to be around to walk my daughters down the aisle one day.

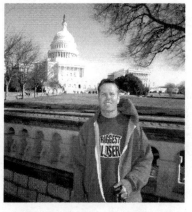

"I started doing what I knew to do. I started exercising and attending a weight loss organization. My brother knew I was attempting to lose weight, so when he heard that the NBC show Biggest Loser was holding auditions locally for teams of two, he asked me if I wanted to go with him. I did. Against all odds, my brother and I were selected to be contestants on season 13 of the show.

"I learned a lot during my time in California filming this reality tv show. A lot of it was good and helpful. However, five and a half months later, the show was over and I went home. I found myself seriously lacking some of the key ingredients that had helped me be successful. I no longer had trainers, nutritionists, and peers that were united with me to help me achieve my goals.

"I set out looking for those who were like-minded as me. People who valued community. People who took a genuine interest in others as they progressed on their own journey. People who valued exercise. People who valued nutrition. People of prayer who included God in their health journey: that was key for me.

"At the beginning of my search for these people, I found Mike and Lillian Smith. What a blessing that was! It was a match made in heaven! They both had a story. They were a wealth of knowledge. They demonstrated extreme wisdom in being able to connect with others and help them get healthier.

"With the help of Mike and Lillian, a community-wide health program began in 2013. It ran for five sessions, and over 1,500 people attended! Those people lost over 15,000 pounds! They also became more flexible! Their cardio improved! Their diets changed! Life-long habits formed!

"I highly recommend Mike and Lillian's new book! The way they weave faith and the way God sees our health with our fitness is masterful! They demonstrate keen insights time and time again! You will definitely want to read this, take notes, and share with your family, friends, and church!"

–Allen "Buddy" Shuh, Pastor & Season 13 Contestant of *Biggest Loser*; Director of the Michigan Chapter of TEARS

"Mike and Lillian have addressed issues of a global health crisis that is rearing its ugly head in evermore profound ways. The gifts that our bodies were intended to be are beginning to turn on us.

"Though scripturally based, this reading is for believers as well as secular thinkers alike. The information here is not only Biblically principled but medically sound/practical.

"Thankfully, they are not just pointing out the problems but offering real world solutions/tools. I encourage everyone/anyone to read this." **– Tommy Aldridge**

World-renowned legendary rock drummer, current member of the rock band Whitesnake (since 1987); Lifelong bike enthusiast and avid road cyclist, logging in hundreds of miles a week even while keeping up with extensive tour schedules

Fit 'n' Faith

LILLIAN EASTERLY-SMITH
& MIKE SMITH

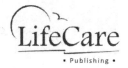

LifeCare
· Publishing ·

Cover design by Kelly Hawkins

ISBN-13: 978-1983470882
ISBN-10: 1983470880

LifeCare Publishing is a branch of
LifeCare Christian Center
A non-profit faith-based ministry
www.LifeCareChristianCenter.org
info.lifecarecc@gmail.com
Westland, MI USA

Mission Statement

LifeCare's mission is to provide opportunities as a care center that offer help, hope and healing in relationships and individually in body, soul and spirit through various resources including counseling, coaching, spiritual direction, classes, transformation groups, seminars, healing weekends and other professional interventions in multiple locations as well as training others to do so worldwide.

CONTENTS

Preface 9

Introduction 11

1 The Why, the What, & the Wait 13

2 Unpacking & Unlearning – Our Story 17

3 Dancing on Glass – the S.A.D. facts (Standard American Diet) 23

4 Necessary Endings & New Beginnings 41

5 Ready, Set, *Grow!* – The Baby Steps 51

6 Weapons of Mass *Distraction* – Staying the Course 71

7 Testimonies & Mess-timonies – Perseverance not Perfection! 85

8 Join the Ant, the Eagle, the Buffalo, and *Us!* 91
   (The freedom of a "Fit 'n' Faith" lifestyle)

9 I love you. I hate you. I need you! 101

10 The Lean Horse Wins the Race! 109

11 30-Day Jumpstart to Healthy Living 123
   Sample Food Plan for 30-Day Jumpstart 138

   APPENDIX: Real Food Recipes 139
               Healing Food Shopping List 205
               Glycemic Index 207
               Feelings Chart 208
               Food Balance Chart 209
               Vegan Proteins 210
               The Ultimate Guide to Nuts 211

CONTENTS

APPENDIX:

        Essential Oils Chart   212

MEET THE AUTHORS   213

ACKNOWLEDGMENTS   217

RESOURCES   219

REFERENCES   221

PREFACE

Ahh, Spring time! If you live in Michigan like we do, the winters are long, cold, and dreary. When Spring finally rolls around it feels like the excitement of Christmas Day all over again. "What is that flaming orange ball in the sky?" is usually a common question of the still-thawing Michiganders. It's wonderful as the snow begins to melt, the flowers start to bloom, and the neighbors watch me in childlike excitement doing cartwheels and back flips. Well, maybe not back flips.

There is one downside to all this seasonal bliss: the dreaded dandelion dilemma! Overnight, they just seem to appear, by the thousands. My unsuccessful method to ridding this rogue group of marauders is usually the same: I mow, mow, mow over and over until they're gone. Well, this lasts about two days, and then they're back again, and they've brought a few hundred friends along for the party. As I come to my senses, I realize the truth is there is only one way to have a healthy, good looking lawn: kill the root. It's that simple – stop cutting off the tops, and just get to the root.

I use this somewhat humorous example to make a point: we must get to the root to make lasting change in our lives. If we don't, then we'll just be cutting off tops and seeing the same crop of "dandelions" re-appear season after season after season. One of the main reasons we wrote this book is to help you begin a brand new season and clear out the weeds that have choked out wholeness and health for so long in so many lives.

Fit 'n' Faith is not only a book of help but of hope – a living hope found in God's Word and what He has provided for us on the earth. We like to call it nature's pharmacy. It will begin to open your eyes and your heart to the *fact* that you *can* have a new and permanent way of living from the inside out. You will hear the heartfelt, uplifting testimonies and (if you will) mess-timonies of those who have embraced the Fit 'n' Faith lifestyle of spirit, soul, and body stewardship.

We intend for this book to not only be a tool for individuals, organizations, and churches, but a movement that will pull many out of the pit they've (oftentimes) been unknowingly pulled into.

Fit 'n' Faith is not meant to be an exhaustive resource of every nook and cranny of wellness, but it is meant to show you a simple step-by-step, bottom shelf, easy way anyone can follow to reap a harvest of benefit from simply doing the right thing consistently over time.

This book was birthed through our own trial and error as God led us to knowledge, people, and places that pulled us up to a new level of living. It is our prayer that you will have ever-increasing wholeness, health, and understanding of God, and that you will learn how to take care of one of the greatest gifts He has given each one of us: His temple – our body.

1 Corinthians 10:31, "So whether you eat or drink, or whatever you do, do it all for the glory of God."

Enjoy the journey!
Mike and Lillian

INTRODUCTION

Fitness and faith in the church should be a beautiful collision that creates a synergy of spirit, mind, and body. But with even a cursory look, we can see that it has become the exact opposite – a head-on collision that has left many a fatality in its wake. Both the legs of food-laden tables and those of weary people in the pews are straining under the weight of what has become the unhealthiest Church in history. This grieves us and the God who made us.

We are filling ourselves to capacity with lavish, calorie-filled delights and processed potluck dinners, all the while glancing right over passages of scripture that are clear about the importance of our bodies, and to whom they truly belong. This pervasive problem has become the new "white elephant" in the sanctuary. We are hoping that providing education, resources, and a plan of action will help make a difference.

Sadly, there are desperate, hurting people standing in long healing lines waiting for that "miracle cure" at the healing service, and then after leaving, wait in even longer lines super-sizing the probable cause of what ails them without even knowing it. Many are deceived, or they just lack the information necessary for change. The deception has led us to become accustomed to eating death and expecting life to arise from it. The

> *The deception has led us to become accustomed*
> *to eating death and expecting life to arise from it.*

Body of Christ is literally limping toward the finish line, out of breath, and barraged with life threatening disease. This should not be! Why is it that we treat our lawn tools and cars better than the most amazing gift He has given us on this earth, *His* temple? We can easily go on a scripture fast for days on end without even thinking about it, but we can't go a day without a Starbucks, McDonalds, or Subway? Again, there are reasons, and we hope to address some of them in this book as well as provide a way out!

2 Corinthians 7:1, "Let us purify ourselves from everything that contaminates spirit and body."

Note: *Fit 'n' Faith* is not suggesting idolizing our bodies, but rather being a good steward of what God calls *very good.* (Genesis 1:31)

1

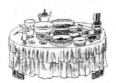

THE WHY, THE WHAT, & THE WAIT

THE "WHY"

1 Corinthians 10:31, "So whether you eat or drink or whatever you do, do it all for the *glory of God*." (*emphasis added*)

This familiar verse is, like many others, often remembered in our head, but never makes its way down to our hearts. Have you ever considered the weight of your "why"? You go to church, go to work, read your devotions, memorize scripture, and, if you're one of the minority of believers, exercise your body on a regular basis. That's all great, but the question is: Why? Is it just because that's what we're told to do? Is your motive aesthetics? Approval? Or is it really for God's glory?

Fit 'n' Faith is, at its core, about the "why" – about what really matters, and about the glory of God – honoring Him in *all* that we are, and in what we do with all He has graciously given us.

We would like to take a bit of creative license with 1 Peter 5:8 (ESV), if you will: "Be sober-minded; be watchful. Your adversary the devil prowls around like a roaring 'LYIN', seeking someone to devour." Friends, you have an enemy, a lying enemy, a fierce foe, who is just as happy if you do nothing at all or you do everything with wrong motives. Either works just as well for his purpose to distract and devour.

If you don't have the right "why", your life will be like a ship with its sail at half-mast. You may get somewhere, but it will be slow. You will most likely be blown off course, and you will end up at the wrong destination. Take some time to examine your "why" and set your sails for God's glory.

THE "WHAT"

What will you do? Free will is the most amazing and potentially dangerous gift God gives. Deuteronomy 30:15-16 (NLT):

> "Now listen! Today I am giving you a choice between life and death, between prosperity and disaster. For I command you this day to love the LORD your God and to keep his commands, decrees, and regulations by walking in his ways. If you do this, you will live and multiply, and the LORD your God will bless you and the land you are about to enter and occupy."

We all make choices every day. How many of them are you making without a second thought? What land are you going to enter today? The land of health or sickness, obedience or rebellion? *You*, and only *you*, get to make that choice.

New beginnings and necessary endings are required to make choices that bring health to spirit and body. The Lord once gave me (Mike) a vision about my choices that has stuck deep in my heart and never left. He showed me a picture of a hot stove, a trash can, and a warm meal on a beautifully set table. The hot stove had a surprisingly sweet-smelling but ugly pot of poison that was boiling over onto the stove. It represented the many choices that if made, would eventually kill me, whether in spirit, mind, or body. The trash was empty. It represented all my current choices that were

14

waste and had to be thrown out so that I could move on to what the Lord wanted for my life. The warm meal on the table was all God was inviting me to that would be healthy for my journey both now and into eternity. The point is this: We all have a hot stove, a trash can, and a warm healthy "meal" to choose from every day of our life. The wonderful truth is that God has provided us His Word, His Spirit, and His Son – more than enough power to make the right choice and enjoy the good results of obedience.

THE "WAIT"

If you put your "but" ☺ before your mind, you will never get out of the starting gate and never experience the wholeness of life. Remember this: We all need to lose *wait!* Excuses are as plentiful as grains of sand on a beach. I would start tomorrow, but…. I would be able to fit it into my schedule, but…… But… But… But. There is a remedy for this, <u>but</u>, it will take faith, trust, and courage.

A friend of mine (Mike) once told me a story about a dream one of his mentors had. It went like this: He was walking on a breezy summer day and became weary, almost to the point of fainting, so he lay down under a very large willow tree and fell fast asleep. He had a dream of what appeared to be a shadow of a figure walking toward him. As the figure got closer, he could tell it was a man. The man began to walk in an aggressive manner, saying louder and louder, "Give me back my stuff!" He didn't know what to make of it and was becoming very fearful. The voice grew even louder and with more authority: "Give me back my stuff!" This happened a third time, so finally the man got up and pleaded, "Please don't harm me; just tell me what stuff I need to give back to you." At that very moment, he realized that this was none other than Jesus Himself. At that instant, His voice softened and He said, "All the stuff that I promised you I would carry and bear so that you could take my light yoke." The man, now in tears, realized that he was carrying all the worry, fear, doubt, shame, and regret that Jesus told him to unload so that he could finish his earthly journey unhindered and fulfilled.

Now is the time to find the right "why", to come to the table for a warm healthy "meal", and unload the excuses that keep you from a beautiful land the Lord wants you to enter.

FIND YOUR "WANT TO's"

It's not the "how to" most of us are missing; it's the "want to". Are the changes we are making really worth the sacrifice? We all have to answer this question. The struggle is partially a lack of healthy self-love and the desire to do self-care. Have you ever heard, "you can't help them unless they want it for themselves"? Or, "they have to want it for themselves; love themselves enough to make the change – get sober – get into recovery – get help"?

Perhaps some of you reading this book can honestly say, "No, I don't love/like myself enough to make any changes at all." YOU are not alone. Most often we have to find external reasons to make significant changes until the internal motivation comes. So, what's your motivation going to be? Here are some ideas. Please take the time to come up with three you can own.

- I want to be alive for my grandkids; not only that, I want to be able to get down on the floor and get back up to play with them.
- I don't want to be a burden to my adult children and end up in a nursing home with some disease.
- I want to be around for my _____'s wedding, graduation, etc.
- I want to be clear-minded and have energy and stamina to do God's work.

We also have to fight against the rationalizations. What are some you have had in the past, or even now? By the way, there is NEVER going to be a perfect time.

Here is a good reminder for all of us:

In Christ – if we want to gain, we have to give up. If we want to be filled, we have to stop filling ourselves – we have to deny ourselves. If we truly want to get close to God, we'll have to distance ourselves from the things that pull us away from Him.

It is always easier to make excuses than to change. What is God calling you to do?

16

2

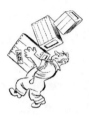

UNPACKING & UNLEARNING

—OUR STORY

My wife, Lillian, seems to adopt a new language or accent on every trip we make, whether near or far. For days after we get home, I still feel like we're in Africa, Mexico, or the good old south, y'all. It usually takes her a day to relearn English and unlearn the native language she has adopted over the past week or so.

Also, when we go on vacation, we usually come back with more than we left with, a lot of which are trinkets that will eventually be put away or given away. It's the same in life, isn't it? We go from place to place, ad to ad, commercial to commercial, influence to influence, collecting misinformation. There are many of these "trinkets" we hang onto our whole life, to our detriment.

Most health journeys are like a trip, ours included. The odd difference is that the health "trip" has, oftentimes, life or death consequences, and yet, it's usually the one we plan for least. Why is it that we plan months ahead for a week vacation, or even a year or two ahead for a wedding, but when it comes to our health and wellness we usually just react, and when sickness comes, we're in shock? We hope, by sharing a portion of our journey, we can help you plan better to make the rest of your years the *best* of your years.

Our journey to wellness has spanned over 11 years. Each step hasn't been a carefully crafted, scientifically researched move forward. Actually, it all started simply enough at a church service as the pastor called for all those with back pain and headaches to come down front for prayers of healing. As we stood watching, a wonderful couple we had just met named Chuck and Sheila stated, "Most of them don't need healing at all; they just need to drink more water." More water for headaches and back pain, really? They went on to explain the natural healing of being fully hydrated and the fact that the vast majority of people are dehydrated. This struck a chord with us, and we started learning a ton from them. Not long after, our church had a seminar with someone who eventually became my (Mike) Chiropractor, Dr. Chris Niedzinski. His wisdom opened up yet another world about healing and wholeness through chiropractic care.

We started devouring books like *Body by God* from Dr. Ben Lerner, and *The China Study* by T. Colin Campbell. We got very serious about health, not just from an external point (although that is good), but from an inner health perspective that included emotional, mental, and spiritual wellness. As we got educated, we figured out we had as much to unlearn as to learn and that ideas have consequences. We had plenty of them embedded in our minds over the years. How many times did we hear, "Milk does a body good", or "Pork, the new white meat"?

The only education most of us have is what I call the "they" knowledge. You know what "they" say seems to be all we know. Who are "they"? Are "they" out for your best? Are "they" lying? Do "they" care about you, or do "they" care about their product and pocket book? These are serious questions that need to be asked – questions that demand an honest answer. You are in a war, my friends.

Take some time to unpack and unlearn. It is critical for you if you want a healthy spiritual and physical future.

UNPACK

What needs to go? Maybe it's the FDA food pyramid, fear of cholesterol and fats, or maybe it's just your own version of the food pyramid. Ask God to reveal what myths and half-truths need to go.

UNLEARN

Do you, like us, have knee-jerk thought reactions when you hear a slogan or catch phrase about faith or fitness? What is it that you must unlearn to move forward with discernment and wisdom?

Be proactive instead of reactive and see how your life can change. It takes a bit of "hard labor" in your mind, but how much more does it take to unlearn than to put the truth in place in the first place? Use every opportunity to learn and grow. The rewards will astound you.

> **The bottom line: John Wooden said, "It's what you learn after you know it all that counts."**

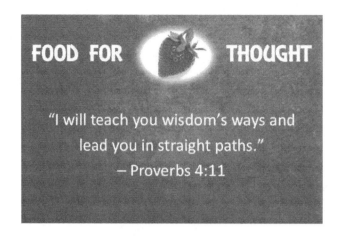

FOOD FOR THOUGHT

"I will teach you wisdom's ways and
lead you in straight paths."
– Proverbs 4:11

Since we shared our story and how the first item of interest to us was water, we want to share a bit about the importance of H_2O.

H_2O – ONE OF THE SIX ESSENTIALS TO LIVING WELL

THE GOAL

Half Your Body Weight in Ounces of GOOD WATER!

For example, if you weigh 180 lbs., your body needs 90 oz. (or roughly 3 quarts) of water each day. If you weigh 120 lbs., you need 60 oz. (or roughly 2 quarts) of water each day.

And what do we mean by good water? Isn't our tap/drinking water good?

Dangers in Your Drinking Water

- Drugs
- Rocket Fuel and Heavy Metals
- Chlorine and Fluoride

As reported in *New Scientist*, a comprehensive survey of U.S. drinking water reveals that your drinking water is likely laced with a wide variety of pharmaceuticals and hormonally active chemicals.

The 11 most frequently detected compounds were:

- **Atenolol**, a beta-blocker used to treat cardiovascular disease
- **Atrazine**, an organic herbicide banned in the European Union which has been implicated in the decline of fish stocks and in changes in animal behavior
- **Carbamazepine**, a mood-stabilizing drug used to treat bipolar disorder
- **Estrone**, an estrogen hormone secreted by the ovaries and blamed for causing gender changes in fish
- **Gemfibrozil**, an anti-cholesterol drug
- **Meprobamate**, a tranquilizer used in psychiatric treatment
- **Naproxen**, a painkiller and anti-inflammatory linked to increases in asthma incidence
- **Phenytoin**, an anticonvulsant used to treat epilepsy
- **Sulfamethoxazole**, an antibiotic
- **TCEP**, a reducing agent used in molecular biology
- **Trimethoprim**, another antibiotic

Tap Water Can Give You Cancer and **Bottled Water is Not the Answer**

And, remember, you can still be exposed to contaminated water when you:
- Shower or bathe
- Wash your hands
- Wash laundry
- Rinse fruits and vegetables
- Wash dishes, glasses, and other utensils

What Should You Do?

Options:

- Bottled Water? NO! Why? Anything in plastic will be high in carcinogens
- Filter on the Tap (ex: PUR – removes impurities but not the chlorine or fluoride)
- Filter on the Shower Head – removes impurities that get absorbed through your skin
- Distiller (1 drawback – it also removes needed minerals, so you will have to supplement)
- Reverse Osmosis – full house vs. countertop (full house filtration system is best but much more costly – if your current budget does not allow the expense, at least get the countertop version)
- Purchase by the Container – many health food stores and even grocery stores have purified water you can purchase by the gallon (feel free to purchase and transport in plastic but store in a glass container when you get home)

Remember:

Lasting Change = a worthy goal + effort + focus

3

DANCING ON GLASS

The S.A.D. Facts (Standard American Diet)

WHAT'S AT STEAK (STAKE)? LIFE-STYLE or LIFE-STIFLE?

Imagine this: You wake up and get set to go for a very long run. You put on a wet pair of Carhartt coveralls and your hiking boots, and then proceed to put 50 lb. weights on top of the boots. If you can even move at all, you probably won't get far, and may even injure yourself. This is kind of a silly, but serious example of the Standard American Diet. Food is meant to be fuel for your body, giving you energy for the journey, just as good, light running shoes and thin clothing are meant to make your run easier and lessen the chance of injury. When we're constantly filling our bodies with super-sized meats, sweets, and carb-laden treats, we are adding the weight that makes our life journey harder, and may just stop it in its tracks long before the finish line.

The majority of Americans have fallen prey to the "SEE food" Diet. Delayed gratification and daily moderation seem to be a thing of the past for a variety of reasons. Most of us are living out the "I want it NOW" mentality, and we have lost the arts and virtues of patience and self-control that lead to wholeness and health. We want immediate relief from discomfort of any sort, so we have played right into the hands of the addictive nature of all humanity. We want a quick fix even after we come to realize how far we have gotten off the path – the path of righteousness and healthy living in all respects. So, we look for the "pill to cure the ill" whether it be emotional, mental or physical. Even spiritually we want a quick fix, so we enter every prayer line, and attend every prayer meeting, Bible study, and conference hoping that God will give instant deliverance so we don't have to do any work.

The wait...just keeps bringing on the weight – there is no change. Perhaps it is time to put "feet to your prayers." We must cooperate with God's leadership and take all that He provides with regard to information/wisdom and apply it to our lives. One of the verses I (Lillian) continue to go back to and share in every class/program we offer is Hosea 4:6, "my people are destroyed from lack of knowledge." We are perishing, being destroyed – it is true, and not only from lack of knowledge, but also from lacking the willingness to live out the truth – apply it. The truth (knowledge) should lead to obedience. And ultimately, it is for our good. God's guidelines/rules/boundaries are ALWAYS for our good.

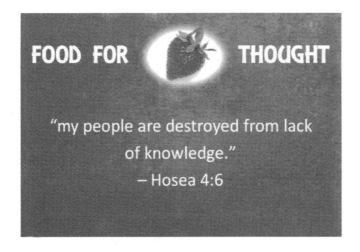

FOOD FOR THOUGHT

"my people are destroyed from lack of knowledge."
– Hosea 4:6

THE S.A.D. (Standard American Diet) LEADS TO OBESITY

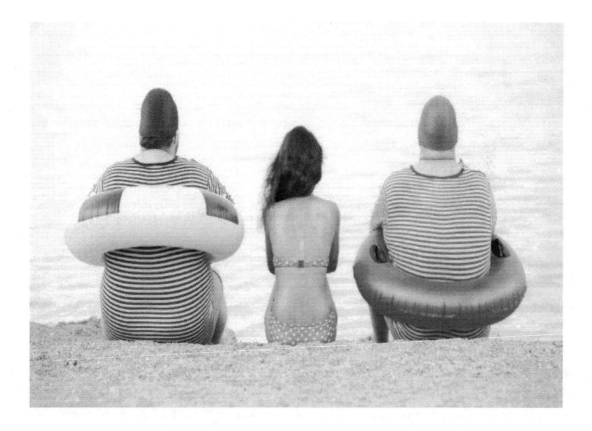

WHAT ARE THE HEALTH CONSEQUENCES OF OBESITY FOR ADULTS?

People who are obese are at increased risk for many diseases and health conditions, including the following:

- All causes of death (mortality)
- High blood pressure (Hypertension)
- High LDL cholesterol, low HDL cholesterol, or high levels of triglycerides (Dyslipidemia)
- Type 2 diabetes
- Coronary heart disease
- Stroke

25

- Gallbladder disease
- Osteoarthritis (a breakdown of cartilage and bone within a joint)
- Sleep apnea and breathing problems
- Chronic inflammation and increased oxidative stress
- Some cancers (endometrial, breast, colon, kidney, gallbladder, and liver)
- Low quality of life
- Mental illness such as clinical depression, anxiety, and other mental disorders
- Body pain and difficulty with physical functioning

- Estimated annual medical cost of obesity in the U.S. was $147 billion in 2008; the medical costs for people who are obese were $1,429 higher than those of normal weight.
- 2/3 of all deaths are lifestyle driven
- 58% of new cases of diabetes can be prevented (CDC/obesity)

THE CAUSE

In 1700, the average individual consumed about 4 pounds of sugar each year.

In 1800, it was about 18 pounds of sugar per year.

In 1900, the average person ate 90 pounds of sugar per year.

In 2009, the average individual consumes 150 pounds per year. Half of our society consumes ½ pound of sugar per day. Most of this is in unnatural, man-made forms such as sucrose and high fructose corn syrup. (Jockers/sugar)

Half of our society consumes ½ pound of sugar per day

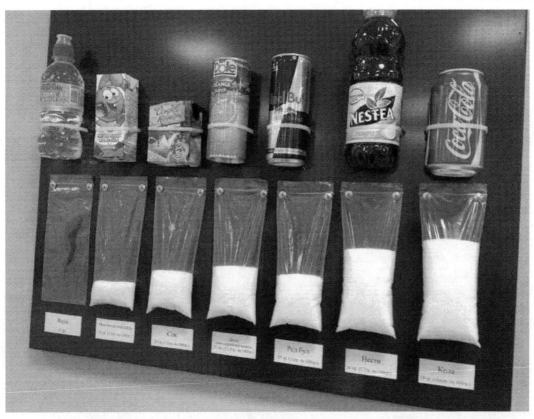

In the image above, the display shows the amount of sugar in each type of drink, with water displayed on the far left and Coca-Cola on the far right.

THE DRUG: SUGAR

- Damages the brain! University of New South Wales concluded chronic sugar intake triggers changes in the area of the brain responsible for memory and stress. (Food Babe/sugar)
- Leads to Type 2 Diabetes, inflammation, high blood pressure, poor sex drive, increased risk of cancer, depression. (Hyman, Dr. Mark/sugar)
- Blood sugar spikes are the enemy of health – cause us to store the extra fuel as fat. Excess fat = toxin storage. (Better Nutrition)

27

- Dr. Joel Kahn, cardiologist: "When my patients go on a sugar detox, we see improvements in blood pressure, cholesterol and blood sugar levels. They feel better – have more energy, a clearing of brain fog, glowing skin and greater calm." (Food Babe/sugar)
- Mayo Clinic warns that sugar is the principal driver of T2 diabetes and heart disease. (Food Babe/sugar)
- 100 grams depresses the immune system (white cell function) by 40% within 30 minutes after ingestion and may last for five hours!!!! (Sears)

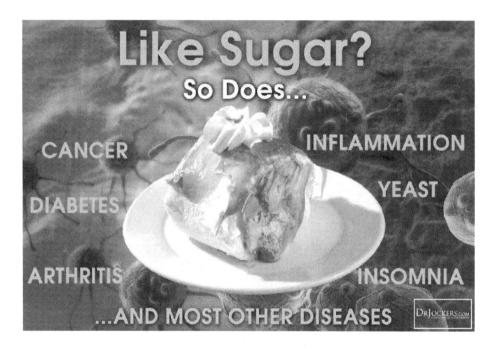

How much is too much?

✓ 7 out of 10 Americans get at least 10% of their daily calories from added sugar.
✓ Those who consume 21% or more of their daily calories in sugar are twice as likely to die from heart disease compared to those who got 7% or less daily. (Mercola/sugar)

So how much should you consume? The American Heart Association recommends:

Recommended Dietary Allowance
FOR SUGAR INTAKE

Category	Age	Amount per day*
Men		9 tsp (38 grams)
Women		6 tsp (25 grams)
Kids	9 & older	Less than 8 tsp (<32 grams)
Kids	4-8 yrs	3 tsp (12 grams)
Kids	under 2 yrs	ZERO (0 grams)

*No more than these amounts.

Sugar is HIGHLY addictive! Some report that it is as addictive as cocaine and affects the same pleasure center of the brain. Here is the cycle:

SUGAR ADDICTION:
THE PERPETUAL CYCLE

1. YOU EAT SUGAR
- You like it, you crave it
- It has addictive properties

2. BLOOD SUGAR LEVELS SPIKE
- Dopamine is released in the brain = addiction
- Mass insulin secreted to drop blood sugar levels

4. HUNGER & CRAVINGS
- Low blood sugar levels cause increased appetite and cravings
- Thus the cycle is repeated

3. BLOOD SUGAR LEVELS FALL RAPIDLY
- High insulin levels cause immediate fat storage
- Body craves the lost sugar "high"

DEALING WITH CRAVINGS (Physically/Body)

FOOD CRAVINGS

YOUR CRAVING	WHAT YOU NEED	WHAT TO EAT INSTEAD
CHOCOLATE	MAGNESIUM	Nuts, seeds, veggies & fruits
SUGARY FOODS	CHROMIUM	Broccoli, grapes, cheese, chicken
	CARBON	Fresh fruits
	PHOSPHORUS	Chicken, beef, fatty fish, eggs dairy, nuts, veggies, grains
	SULPHURE	Cranberries, horseradish, cabbage, cauliflower
	TRYPTOPHAN	Cheese, raisins, sweet potatoes, spinach
BREAD, PASTA & OTHER CARBS	NITROGENE	High protein foods: meat, fatty fish, nuts, beans, chia seeds
OILY FOODS	CALCIUM	Organic milk, cheese, green leafy vegetables
SALTY FOODS	CHLORIDE	Fatty fish, goat milk
	SILICON	Cashews, nuts, seeds

Source: Coaching & Weight Management

stepintomygreenworld.com

DEALING WITH CRAVINGS (Emotionally/Mentally)

Uncover your sugar triggers – What draws you to sugar?
- Reward?
- Social?
- Stress?
- Grief?
- That time of the month?

Choose something new – a new coping mechanism! Here are a few ideas:

Things To Do When You're Feeling Down

Nurture Yourself
Drink a cup of hot tea
Wear soft comfortable clothes
Take a bubble bath
Take a long shower
Get a massage
Get a manicure
Read a magazine
Wash your hair
Wrap up in a blanket
Give yourself a facial
Color in a coloring book
Play with Play Doh
Blow bubbles
Light candles
Read a children's book
Make a snack
Take a nap
Sing / Listen to music
Sit in the sun
Watch a funny video
Watch a good movie
Read a joke book
Watch the clouds go by
Play with a pet
Drive with windows down
Braid your hair

Engage Your Brain
Do a crossword puzzle
Research a topic
Complete a maze
Play a word game
Organize something
Listen to a teaching on CD or YouTube
Write a story
Learn a new skill
Visit a bookstore or library
Plan something
Read a good book
Journal

Move
Take a walk
Wash dishes
Stretch
Dance in your living room
Iron some clothes
Plant something
Go to a park
Cook a nice meal
Dust the living room
Buy flowers
Drive to a new town
Hula hoop
Jump rope
Play basketball
Do an exercise video
Jog around the block
Cut the grass
Play tennis
Rearrange your house
Swim
Do water aerobics
Walk through a sprinkler
Walk at the mall
Wash your sheets
Ride a bike
Take karate lessons
Weed the garden
Go bowling

Be Social
Call a friend
Make a gift for someone
Write a thank you card
Write a letter or note
Meet a friend for lunch
Visit a nursing home
Counsel someone
Give some money away
Organize a card game
Invite someone shopping
Bake bread for a neighbor
Send an encouraging email

Get Creative
Doodle
Invent something
Paint
Play an instrument
Draw
Create a video
Draw a cartoon
Create a new outfit
Visit an art museum
Go to the symphony
Do a craft project
Create a new recipe
Write a song or poem
Cook a new dish
Decorate your house
Knit / Sew / Crochet
Paint a piece of furniture

Be Spiritual
Attend a church service
Read the Bible
Memorize a Bible verse
Listen to worship music
Watch worship online
Pray
Meditate on a Bible verse
Listen to a sermon online
Pray with friends
Visit a Christian bookstore
Attend a Bible study
Pray in a church building
Organize a prayer meeting

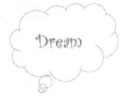

Dream

THE SOLUTION

- I will work toward balancing my life (body, soul, spirit).
- Rely on the Lord. Seek His help and power. Zechariah 4:6, "Not by might nor power, but by MY Spirit says the LORD." (*emphasis added*)
- Run from quick fixes! Diets don't work and neither does some pill or powder.
- Give ALL of you to God – Daily! See Romans 12:1-2
- Keep your goals readily available and in mind.

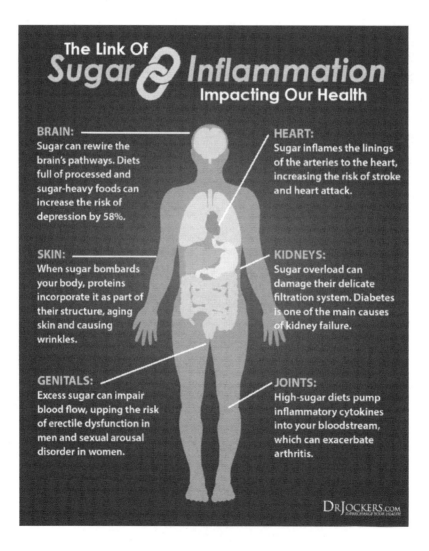

INFLAMMATION

Another consideration for limiting the intake of sugar is inflammation (which leads to pain and discomfort as well as many inflammatory diseases). Inflammation, however, also has another source. It is caused from a highly acidic environment in the body. What people don't know is that meat is one of the culprits, and to add to it, meat is much harder to digest than fruits and vegetables. The S.A.D. includes far more meat and meat products than we really need or can handle. For this reason, we encourage people to begin to cut back on animal proteins. The following gives you all the up-to-date information on protein that will help you sort through the reductions you need to make.

PROTEIN

How Much Daily Protein Do We Really Need?

The Food and Nutrition Board of the Institute of Medicine recommends:

Children:
Age 1-3   13 grams per day
Age 4-8   19 grams per day
Age 9-13   34 grams per day
Age 14-18   46 grams per day

Recommended Dietary Allowance
FOR PROTEIN INTAKE FOR CHILDREN

Age	Grams per day
1-3	13
4-8	19
9-13	34
14-18	46

The recommended dietary allowance (RDA) for adults is 0.8 grams of protein for each kilogram of body weight, regardless of age. This looks like:

- An adult male who is not an avid, marathon-type of exerciser, will need 56 grams of daily protein.
- An adult female who is not an avid, marathon-type of exerciser will need 46 grams of protein daily.
- A pregnant or lactating woman's daily protein intake should be 71 grams.
- Men over age 50, who are less efficient in using amino acids for muscle protein synthesis should have a daily intake of protein of at least 56 grams; however, researchers from the University of Arkansas Department of Geriatrics found that going above the RDA is particularly beneficial for seniors. As published in the 2008 "Clinical Nutrition" journal, researchers noted that getting 1.5 grams of protein for each kilogram of body weight can improve health. This higher recommendation may boost immune health, aid in wound healing, help control blood pressure and even keep your bones as strong as possible.
- Women over age 50 should strive for at least 46 grams; however, more is desirable for the reasons stated above.

Recommended Dietary Allowance
FOR PROTEIN INTAKE FOR ADULTS

Adult	Grams per day
Average male	56
Average female	46
Pregnant/Lactating women	71
Men over 50	56+
Women over 50	46+

Why Do We Need Protein?

Protein is considered a macronutrient, which means that your body needs it in large amounts every day to function properly. When you eat protein, your body breaks it down into amino acids that are used for several purposes. Protein can provide your body with energy when necessary, but you should not rely on protein as a primary energy source because it has more important physiological roles to play, according to "Nutrition and You" by Joan Salge Blake.

Your immune system relies heavily on proteins. When your body is exposed to potentially harmful substances, such as bacteria or a virus, your immune system sends out proteins called antibodies. These antibodies seek out and attack the virus or bacterium in an attempt to neutralize it and prevent it from multiplying and causing illness.

Your bodily fluids – blood, saliva, etc. – function best at a neutral pH, or approximately 7.0. [You can purchase PH paper to test your levels to keep them in balance at any health food store – it is similar to testing pH for a swimming pool. Consider this: what would happen if you never balanced PH levels in a pool? That should give you a good picture of why it is important to keep our bodies in balance.] Many things that you encounter daily, such as foods, beverages and pollution, can change the pH of bodily fluids. A drastic and persistent change in pH can lead to chronic symptoms and various health problems. The proteins in your body act as buffers that help keep your pH neutral. When the pH of your blood becomes too acidic, the protein buffers in the blood will pick up hydrogen ions until the pH returns to neutral. If the pH becomes too high, or basic, protein buffers release hydrogen ions to lower the pH.

There is protein in every single cell in your body – from your hair to your nails to your muscles and organs. These proteins are known as structural proteins; they quite literally provide the structure for your body. Without them, you could not walk, run or even stand. In fact, the most abundant protein in your body is collagen, which is present in skin, ligaments, tendons and bones.

Proteins also play a vital role in nutrient transport. They carry sodium and potassium into and out of cells in order to maintain the proper electrolyte balance. Proteins also carry vitamins, such as vitamin A, from your organs to your cells. A specific protein in your red blood cells, hemoglobin, is responsible for carrying oxygen from your lungs to your cells. Hemoglobin also takes carbon dioxide from your cells to your lungs, so that it can be expelled from the body. (Healthy Eating)

What is the Difference Between Plant and Animal Protein?

The primary difference between animal and plant proteins is their amino acid profiles, and it is those profiles that direct the rates at which the absorbed amino acids are put to use within the body. Animal-based proteins, of course, are much more similar to our proteins, thus are used more readily and rapidly than plant proteins. That is, "substrate" amino acids derived from animal-based proteins are more readily available for our own protein synthesizing reactions which allows them to operate at full [capacity]. Plant proteins are somewhat compromised by their limitation of one or more amino acids. When we restore the relatively deficient amino acid in a plant protein, we get a response rate equivalent to animal proteins. [T. Colin Campbell's] lab produced experimental data to support this view – and of course, similar observations of years past in other laboratories can also been interpreted in this way. (Campbell)

What Foods Have Complete Protein?

"A complete protein (or whole protein) is a source of protein that contains an adequate proportion of all nine of the essential amino acids necessary for the dietary needs of humans" and some other animals. (Wikipedia/Complete Protein)

Here are several healthy and complete proteins you can add to your daily food plan:

- Quinoa — 8 grams per one cup serving, cooked
- Buckwheat — 6 grams per one cup serving, cooked
- Hempseed — 10 grams per 2 Tablespoon serving
- Chia Seeds — 4 grams per 2 Tablespoon serving
- Rice and Beans — 7 grams per one cup serving
- Ezekiel Bread — 8 grams per 2-slice serving
- Hummus and Pita — 7 grams per 1 whole-wheat pita and 2 Tablespoons of hummus
- Spirulina with grains or nuts — 4 grams per 1 Tablespoon

It is nearly impossible to ever become deficient in protein.

Here is a short list of veggies that you can easily include in your daily diet and the subsequent amount of protein in each.

- Spouted beans, peas and lentils – 4.6 grams per ½ cup
- Green peas – 11.6 grams per cup
- Kale – 0.7 grams per cup
- Collard greens – 1.1 grams per cup

- Pinto, garbanzo, white, kidney, lima and soy beans – The average protein content of beans is 9 grams per 100 grams (about ½ cup). Some varieties contain as much as 12 grams per 100 grams.
- Brussels sprouts – 2 grams per ½ cup
- Asparagus – over 3 grams per cup
- Raw cauliflower – 2 grams per cup
- Raw broccoli – 2.6 grams per cup
- Artichoke, one – over 4 grams
- Squash, Hubbard cooked – 5.1 grams per cup
- Spinach, cooked – over 5 grams per cup
- One large russet potato – 8 grams of protein

If you consumed just these in one day, look at how much protein you would consume!

Asparagus 3g	Spinach 5g
Cauliflower 2g	Potato 8g
Broccoli 2.6g	Beans 9g
Artichoke 4g	

Total 33.6g

Kids are in far greater danger of not getting adequate vitamin D, omega 3s and B-12 than they are protein.

As Dr. Joel Furhman states, "It is almost impossible to not get enough protein unless the diet is deficient in calories." 10 to 15% of calories in the form of protein will be ample.

Most vegan adults get 60 to 80 grams of protein daily – more than ample. Children will get less according to age/weight.

So, when people ask you, "Where do you get your protein?" Don't worry; you've got a rock-solid answer now. (Myhdiet/protein)

Here's what to look for to tell if you're lacking in protein

Heather Crosby, vegan nutritional expert and a T. Colin Campbell Foundation Certified Plant-Based Wellness Coach, says to look for the following signs if you're worried about protein deficiency:

- Anxiety/Depression (amino acids fuel the neurotransmitters serotonin and dopamine that prevent depression and anxiety)
- Poor injury recovery (protein fuels muscle recovery and regrowth)
- Hair Loss/Breakage (protein supports collagen production in the hair, skin, and nails)
- Inability to focus (amino acids support brain performance)
- Constant muscle pain (protein helps muscle recovery and aids in repair)
- Brittle/Breaking nails (protein supports collagen production in the hair, skin, and nails)
- Poor muscle tone, even with exercise (protein builds and maintains lean muscle mass)
- Constantly fatigued (protein is needed for a healthy metabolism)
- Digestive issues (protein aids in digestion)

It's important to note that a diet too low in calories or too high in sugar will also cause these symptoms, so eliminate those causes before you add more protein.

Most people only need 0.5 grams of protein per pound of body weight to maintain lean muscle mass, but could eat up to 1 gram of protein per pound of body weight to gain lean muscle.

Now you can relax: a diet rich in whole foods will give your muscles all the protein you could dream of. (One Green Planet)

- See Appendix for Vegan Protein Chart

4

NECESSARY ENDINGS
& NEW BEGINNINGS

AIR BRUSH, HAIR BRUSH, AND THE FULL-LENGTH MIRROR –
Holly*weird's* Identity Theft Scam

Modern day living has us constantly adjusting to what is beautiful, healthy, or pleasing. By the world's standard, we can't keep up with the never-ending barrage of the "who's who" of the fashion, entertainment, or sports world. The latest and greatest new spiritual revelation or health discovery promises to make you feel good about yourself or give you the fountain of youth, energy, and look that you've always wanted. "Hollyweird" has deceived many a mind into thinking their standard is truth—the way it should be. Is their "truth" *really* beauty? Is it *really* true health? Or, is it just the creation of a veneer that covers up what needs to be changed from within?

How much computer enhancement did it take to make that person on the magazine cover look that way? It probably took a lot longer than it took for the photo shoot itself. Facebook can easily turn into "fakebook" and cause a quick slide down into the comparison trap as well. When we look at our own life, it seems to be as if we have a funhouse mirror in front of us; everything looks disfigured and bizarre. You are not Hollywood or Facebook. These comparisons have helped cause depression and insecurity for so many, as well as a loss of hope. Remember this: You are God's masterpiece, made just the way He planned. You don't need to bear the image of anyone else. You are one of a kind. Psalm 139:13-14 is a solid, unchanging truth about what real beauty is all about:

> [13] You made all the delicate, inner parts of my body and knit them together in my mother's womb. [14] Thank you for making me so wonderfully complex! It is amazing to think about. Your workmanship is marvelous—and how well I know it. (TLB)

Your uniqueness, not conformity, is what God wants you to work on. This being said, we want you to be the best you, you can be. That is why we focus more on lifestyle change than losing weight. If you make good choices and change your lifestyle, however, the byproduct will be weight loss which is a good thing if you need to lose a few pounds.

Think about being at a rest stop or a mall and you are trying to find a location. There is always an X or a dot that says, "you are here." Your life says this as well. You *are* here, and you can't be anywhere else right now, and that's ok. There is a "there" you should be striving to get to, but not by comparison or by external obsession. Romans 12:2 tells us, "Do not conform to the pattern of this world, but be transformed by the renewing of your mind. Then you will be able to test and approve what God's will is—his good, pleasing and perfect will." God's will is that we take care of all of who we are and the gifts He has given us.

I'm always reminded of what one of my (Mike) heroes of the faith, Dr. Charles Stanley, says: "Do your best, look your best, and be your best." Notice he said *your,* not *their* best. You are an amazing, one of a kind, spectacular creation, **period**, so get used to it. ☺

A fancy wrapper is nice, but what is on the inside is what really counts. The truth is: when the inside is healthy, the outside will follow. Sometimes we get disappointed with how far we've let ourselves go. This can actually be a great motivation. By reframing our perception, we can turn this into a positive. You may be a mess right now, but you're still a beautiful mess. There are so many physical and spiritual qualities we have right now that we can thank God for. Spend some time writing/listing some of these qualities and keep them in a place where you can see them, so when the enemy brings Hollyweird or Fakebook to your mind or eyes, you don't have to compare yourself to anyone but wonderful you.

Bad Carrots?

Have you ever eaten a rotten vegetable? Nothing tastes quite like it. Sometimes they look great on the outside, but on the inside, they are decayed and diseased. And...you've heard the dangling carrot expression, right? Each day there are many "carrots" hanging before us bidding us to come and "eat." We've mentioned a few, but there are many more that are cleverly disguised. Comparison to a make-believe world is low hanging fruit with a very high price tag. We suggest that it may be time for a fast of some kind – perhaps it is time for a fast from media images for a season, or even permanently. You don't need "them" to tell you what beauty is, you just need a mirror and the truth of God.

With all this being said, we want you to move forward with confidence and set some goals that make the best you possible. Take the time to evaluate where you are and where you want to be in the next few months. Break it down – next 3 months, 6 months, and then a year from now. How can you be the best "you" you can be? Perhaps the following chapters will help you do just that. We believe it is important to write it down and also seek out some accountability!

> *Move forward with confidence and set some goals that make the best you possible.*

WEARY OF PAIN AND PLEASURE

"Most of us don't mind doing what we ought to do when it doesn't interfere with what we want to do, but it takes discipline and maturity to do what we ought to do whether we want to or not." – Joseph B. Wirthlin

In this chapter, through questions, contemplating, and time alone with God, we want you to take an aerial look at your life and habits and dig in deep to see what is of value to your quest for wholeness and quality of life both now and in the future. This is a needed cleansing process that will free you to move forward and get beyond the starting gate stage.

Comedian Steven Wright once said, "You can't have it all, where would you put it?" Humorous, yes, but oh, so true. We can't have it all, do it all, or be it all—there's just no room. We need to find out what is not working, what is a "garage sale" item we're hanging onto, and what needs to be replaced in order to make wiser choices for our journey.

You're Fired!

You really ought to end some things. Really!

"One of the most important types of decision-making is deciding what you are *not* going to do, what you need to eliminate in order to make room for strategic investments." – Dr. Henry Cloud

We can compare this to the super-sizing food gimmick the fast food chains have used for years. You get *all* this food for just a few pennies more. Yes, you get all the fake food, but your body and brain are looking for nutrition to run on, so they call for more food, and then you go back again and again. More calories with less nutrition is the truth of the matter. If you want health, you have to stop super-sizing your life with a "junk food" agenda and start trimming down to get the nutrient life. Keep more "vegetables" on your "plate of life" – having *more* and *"all"* just doesn't work. Tell those extras, you're fired! Starting today!

You're Hired!

Growing companies are always looking for good vibrant employees who will bring value to their organization. Wise hiring includes getting the right person on the right seat on the right bus, so to speak. If a company just wants to fill space and get as many hired as possible, they will fail in short order.

You are the CEO of "Your Life, Inc." You choose who you want to hire. Be wise and hire lean, mean, go-getters who will not just take up space, but will be able to make

"Your Life, Inc." flourish and be a well-oiled machine that will prosper for the long haul. What questions will you ask potential hires? Are you experienced? Prompt? Honest?

Many leadership teachers remind us that when we are starting, we need to keep the end in mind, and that advice is extremely wise. We would like to suggest something to go along with that advice. End with the beginning in mind. So many of us get excited about stopping a habit, ending a toxic relationship, or leaving a job that has no future that we just stop there and then look around wondering what to do, what is next? When you think about ending, think about beginning or you might just find yourself like a little child who's just lost his mother at the mall.

So, you say you're not sure what to end or begin – here are some suggestions that might be helpful:

Look at your Calendar, your Cupboard, your Desk, and your Closet
Find the excess or scarcity that needs to be addressed. Be brutally honest with yourself here. Some things are toxic and we still hang onto them. Why? Even "yuckiness" is better than the unknown in our minds. I recall financial expert, Dave Ramsey, saying something to this effect concerning toxic debt: he used the example of a baby in a dirty diaper. "I know it smells bad, but it's warm and it's mine!" Graphic example, yes, but now you get the point.

Take the time right now to list the things you will begin and the things you will end.

1.

2.

3.

4.

5.

"It takes a lot of energy when we have excess, and a lot of faith for a new beginning, but when one is fired and then another is hired, you will be free." – Mike Smith

This practice will open time and opportunity to live life with purpose and wisdom. You will be able to, as leadership expert Michael Hyatt says, "Manage your energy, not your time." Very wise counsel from someone who lives out this principle.

D.W.I.N. (Deal With It Now)

Our DWIN method has saved us countless hours of second guessing and dealing with regret. If you have to end or begin something, deal with it now! There is a phenomenon called "analyzation paralyzation" that happens when we put off what we know needs to end or begin. Many do this all the time. We know it's time to take some action, but we let fear or just plain laziness keep us from it. Sadly, we rarely think about the future or possible consequences when we're in this state. What do you want your spiritual, emotional, mental, and physical health to look like next month, year, five years from now? It is crucial that you answer this. The quality and quantity of your life depends on it. Ask God to reveal any hidden areas of your life that need to be addressed now.

It's Time to Lose Some *Wait!*

Make a list of the D.W.I.N. questions you need to ask yourself below.

1.

2.

3.

4.

5.

Psalm 118:24 (ESV), "This is the *minute, day, year, and life* the Lord has made; let us rejoice and be glad in it." *(emphasis added)* Remember, one of the most dangerous words we can speak about changing our life is: *tomorrow.*

Now that you've made your lists, we want you to take a close look at them and narrow them even further. We live in the age of excessive options and information. Take a silent retreat and seek God to give you revelation of His will, and ask Him to let you see what truly is the right path to take. God won't reveal ten different paths and confuse you like Google will. He will direct you according to His way and the way He specifically wired you. It's okay to look at your life and say honestly, "This activity, relationship, job, hobby, really drains me and I don't want it anymore." It's also okay to say, "This really fills me, and if it is within the guidelines of God's Word, I want more of it." Remember, what fills you will give you more to give away to others; what drains you will take energy and time away from your purpose and your potential to bless others.

"THE" Necessary Ending

We all have an unknown "expiration date" on our birth/death certificate. Either the Lord will come back, or we will go to Him when He comes back like "a thief in the night."

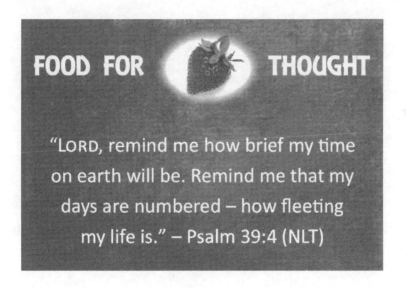

FOOD FOR THOUGHT

"LORD, remind me how brief my time on earth will be. Remind me that my days are numbered – how fleeting my life is." – Psalm 39:4 (NLT)

Spiritually – Ask God to give you the desire to be healthy and the strength to follow through on what He asks you to do. If you're not willing, say this prayer: "God help me become willing. Amen!" Step 3 in the 12-step program is all about surrender. We must turn our lives and our wills over to God – let HIM be in control – even in this area of our lives.

Physically – Turn your spiritual insights into practical choices as God leads and directs you "one day at a time." Admit your issues and do something about it – hypertension, low energy, overweight, achy, getting sick more often, have the onset of some disease?

Mentally – Delete "com" from compromise and start with a promise. We were made for more than compromise. We were made for God's promises – in EVERY area of our lives!!! Look for the promises in His Word, and cling to them with regard to your needs and other areas of your life. Begin to change your thinking – "be transformed by the renewing of your mind." (Romans 12:2)

Emotionally – Just like any area of recovery and/or growth, we have to "feel, deal & heal." We can no longer eat or "not eat" to suppress or control our emotions. We MUST learn healthy ways of expressing and releasing them.

Let's go a little bit deeper about the topic of emotions and how to get emotional health that prevents physical un-health.

HOW YOUR EMOTIONS AFFECT YOUR BODY

Here are just a few ways in which specific emotions affect specific bodily functions:

A University of Arizona study found that expressing affectionate feelings towards your loved ones can lower cholesterol.

A study published in the International Journal of Psychophysiology discovered that when subjects simply recalled the situation that had been the initial cause of stress, their blood pressure rates raised significantly. Another study at the University of Maryland Medical Center found that just the anticipation of laughter began to reduce the stress hormones cortisol and adrenaline.

A study at Loma Linda University in California found that when individuals laughed at a funny movie, the levels of beta-endorphins, responsible for mood elevation, rose as well. In addition, Human Growth Hormone, which aids in sleep and contributes to cellular repair, rose by 87%. (TTAC/emotions)

Emotional Clearing for Better Health (Edited from an article published by *The Truth About Cancer*)

Clearing emotions and managing stress go hand in hand. Before you can truly clear emotions, you must learn how to manage stress in order to get cortisol levels down. There is a direct and proven correlation between chronically high cortisol levels (i.e., chronic stress) and cancer.

Here are four basic things you can do NOW to manage stress, lower cortisol levels, and clear stressful emotions so that true healing can occur:

1. **Reflect on what keeps you stressed in your life and DECIDE to make a change.** Divorce, the death of a loved one, finances, even happy occasions like getting married can add to the stress factor. A major source of on-going stress for many Americans is work-related. An Oxford Health Plans study found that 1 in 5 Americans will go to work even if they are ill, injured, or seeing a doctor that day. Reflect on what is causing you stress right now. On a scale from one to ten, how would you rate this stress? Decide if you want this number to go down. Then make a commitment to yourself and your health by determining to make a positive change towards lower stress overall.

2. **Consider tried and true modalities to manage stress**. Once you have decided to lower stress and clear emotions for health, decide on some modalities that will help you get there! Consider Inner Healing Prayer, reflexology, massage, chiropractic care, meditation, prayer, journaling, exercise, and eating healthier. These are all things you can do STARTING NOW to lower stress responses and add a little more self-care to your life. Remember that self-care equals emotional care! And you don't have to do them all. Simply choose one or two modalities, then give it a try. Even taking 10 minutes on your lunch break for a leisurely stroll can sometimes do the trick.

3. **Don't go it alone.** Study after study has shown that those who have the support of a caring group of loved ones have a better chance of coming out of a cancer diagnosis than those who "go it alone." And according to Lissa Rankin, MD, "Individuals who

attend religious services regularly live 7.5 years longer than those who never or rarely attend religious gatherings." So whether it is a church group, a cancer support group, or a group of loving friends, make a list of who you want on your "Healing A-Team" and then get the help and support that you need!

4. **Don't be afraid to "sit" with your emotions**. As we begin to take a break from the "24/7 stress fest" and begin to make room for reflection and healing, it is natural for deeper issues, memories, or events to rise to the surface. Emotions may come out of nowhere, and this is very normal. Practice sitting with emotions as they rise to the surface, and always remember that no matter how bad you may feel, these emotions are coming up to be released. They won't last forever. In fact, there is a good chance that you will feel better after the tears come and go! Studies have found that emotional tears contain high numbers of stress hormones and neurotransmitters, leading researchers to conclude that crying is one way that the body removes stress chemicals. (TTAC/emotions)

...always remember that no matter how bad you may feel, these emotions are coming up to be released. They won't last forever.

5

READY, SET, *GROW!*

The Baby Steps

MOVE FORWARD!

"If you can't fly, run. If you can't run, walk. If you can't walk, crawl, but by all means, keep moving." – Dr. Martin Luther King, Jr.

Physically and spiritually, your life is like going up a down escalator; if you stop, you start going backwards. Why? Your physical and spiritual health can't remain neutral. Once you stop feeding yourself with viable nutrition for the soul and body, it remains hungry and will take whatever the world wants to hand out just to get a quick fix.

Try putting down your Bible or stop going to church for a couple of weeks and see the change that transpires. The media has a tasty smorgasbord of "mind dumbing and numbing" for you to try 24/7. "Mickey D's" says, "Come on down, we have 'happy meals' for a little over a dollar." Never mind that this isn't REAL food, or that our vast array of chemicals has the potential of shortening your life; just come on and be "satisfied" now.

If you want to be physically and spiritually fit, you can't get there in neutral. Picture this if you want to be static in either: You are on a tall stool and you're having a tug-of-war with a very strong person who is on the ground. Who is going to win? It will always be the one on the ground trying to pull you down. The one on the ground is your *enemy!* Back to Martin Luther King's statement: Move forward!!

The Old Way Has to Go

Ephesians 4:17-24 (MSG, *paraphrased*) says,

17-19 And so I insist—and God backs me up on this—that there be no going along with the crowd, the empty-headed, mindless crowd. They've refused for so long to deal with God that they've lost touch not only with God but with reality itself. They can't think straight anymore. Feeling no pain, they let themselves go in sexual obsession, addicted to every sort of perversion.

20-24 But that's no life for you. You learned Christ! My assumption is that you have paid careful attention to him, been well instructed in the truth precisely as we have it in Jesus. Since, then, we do not have the excuse of ignorance, everything—and I do mean everything—connected with that old way of life has to go. It's rotten through and through. Get rid of it! And then take on an entirely new way of life—a God-fashioned life, a life renewed from the inside and working itself into your conduct as God accurately reproduces his character in you.

We are all a bundle of desires, both old and new. The "old spirit/physical man" loves spiritual and physical "junk food": lies, lust, greed, fries, candy, pop, etc. The "new man" needs new food: purity, love, truth, veggies, fruit, etc. Old food disintegrates and dissolves health; new food nourishes and brings life. Even old harmless things eventually turn ruinous. Why? They all have the enticement of the enemy's concealing character:

Lies! He (Satan) was a liar from the start. A reinvention that comes from the inside out is what we can have in God. He wants His character infused in your life.

Don't fear. You won't grow and learn without stumbling a bit. Don't expect a perfect "repentance" of the old ways. No matter how carefully we plan, we will at some point stagger a bit, or more than a bit. Hang in there! Do not give up when you stumble!

The Key: Walk, then Run!

My (Mike) sister and brother-in-law had four very "active" boys who tried to run long before they got walking down to a fine art. They were at our house just about every weekend, and on countless occasions, one or more would get hurt, sometimes requiring stitches. Why? RUNNING!! Our coffee table was a forehead magnet for these ambitious, young house-Olympians. Trips to the emergency room were plentiful and interrupted many a fine meal.

What happens when we try to go too fast, whether that be in faith (spiritually) or fitness (physically/bodily)? We trip and fall, and occasionally receive "stitches" in order to mend the injury. Physically we can trip back into old habits. Spiritually, when we don't have a solid foundation in the Word, we can fall into temptation and false teachings. Both are danger zones that can lead to disaster on down the line.

A few years ago, we came across the 1% living principle. Even if you change a habit just 1% a day, in just over three months you can completely renew or revitalize your life. This is a great way to prevent tripping and falling – one step at a time, one day at a time.

GO, CHRIS, GO!

As a young man, I (Mike) loved to roller skate. In particular, I loved speed skating. I marveled at the speed skating team that I always wanted to be a part of. They were all amazing skaters, but one was kind of a hero to me. His name was Chris. He was the pace setter. He wasn't the quickest or most agile, but he was solid, steady, and had stamina. He would set the pace for a few laps and then the others would tear it up from there until the end.

How are you setting your pace? Do you have one?

Who or what is your pacesetter? Is it the world? The media? Your family?

Don't fear if you don't grow and learn without flaw. FACT: You will not have a perfect "repentance" of the old ways, and that's okay. It's actually a good thing because it can keep us humble and reaching up to God for help. We like to call these: "valleys of sanctification." When you are in one, learn from it and let it be an opportunity for growth. Setbacks can be the catalyst for a more solid foundation of faith, as well as other areas of our lives.

Here is a "Sanctification Valley" example: You've gone three months without sugar and decide that you're now strong enough to nibble on a tasty tidbit at your best friend's wedding. Then, boom! It seems like out of nowhere you go on a week-long sugar binge, pounding your pancreas and sending your insulin levels into outer space.

A quick look at Hebrews 11 (often referred to as the Heroes of Faith chapter), and we see this struggling, failing, reaching, and hoping cycle. Valleys of sanctification are growth opportunities and they can give hope (of what is not yet seen). Your future of faith and fitness is not yet seen. This is exciting news! You can help the outcome by what you do now. In Hebrews 11, the "heroes" didn't get all that was promised in this world. This is actually good for us to think about and consider, because we can look forward to the better health, and the FAR better country, which is our REAL home. We're here to steward what we have, and by faith, move forward to the next life stage.

You can actually take the life stages of personhood and apply them to any area of your life. Whatever life stage you're currently in, keep moving forward. There is much unseen wholeness to strive for.

- Breast Feeding Stage: At this stage you need constant nutrients from another source. You are not able to feed yourself yet.
- Baby Formula Stage: You're able to take in more solid nutrients, tolerate more calories, etc.
- Solid Food Stage: Now you can get foods that are conducive for growth at a faster rate.
- Growth Spurt Stage: All the baby steps have paid off and you are growing steadily.

- Adolescence Stage: This is where good risk-taking starts and moves you into a flow of wholeness.
- Adulthood Stage: You are now mature and know what works and what doesn't. You have the wisdom and experience to stay whole.
- Golden Years Stage: You reap all the benefits of each step of growth, and if an obstacle should arise, you have the power to persevere and recover.

THE BOTTOM LINE

SPIRITUAL – Systematically read and learn God's Word so that you'll be able to weed out all the spiritual junk food the world may be offering you.

PHYSICAL – Apply the baby steps in all areas of your life so that you build a solid foundation and don't leave the path to wholeness.

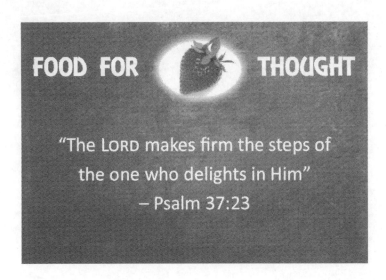

FOOD FOR THOUGHT

"The LORD makes firm the steps of the one who delights in Him"
– Psalm 37:23

BABY STEPS OVERVIEW

Following is the Baby Step Plan we have put together for you. As you slowly make changes, they will become a way of life and not a "temporary" behavior. But before we go into the actual plan, we would like to highlight a few tidbits that will be addressed there and in the other programs we offer.

We mention the importance of detoxification in our classes, in the Baby Step Program, as well as the 30-Day Jumpstart Plan, and we believe the old slogan "a picture is worth a thousand words." Why do we need to buy more organic? Why do we need to detox? This picture explains it. Any questions?

CONVENTIONAL STRAWBERRY

ORGANIC STRAWBERRY

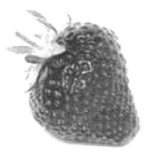

LIVE LOVE FRUIT

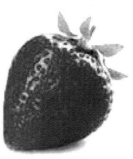

Ingredients: Capton, Pyraclostrobin, Boscalid, Tetrahydrophthalimide, Myclobutanil, Pyrimethanil, Fludioxonil, Bifenthrin, Malathion, Fenhexamid, Cyprodinil, Carbendazim, Malaoxon, Azoxystrobin, Methomyl, Quinoxyfen, Fenpropathrin, Acetamiprid, Propiconazole, Bifenazate, Thiamethoxam, Spinosad A, Methoxyfenozide, Triflumizole, Dichlorvos, Hexythiazox, Metalaxyl, Propiconazole II, Thiabendazole, Spinosad D, Imidacloprid, Endosulfan sulfate, Propiconazole I, Iprodione, Piperonyl butoxide, Endosulfan II, Chlorpyrifos, Carbaryl, Pyriproxyfen, Endosulfan I, 1-Naphthol, Acephate, Clothianidin, Azinphos methyl, Naled, Cyhalothrin, Dicloran, Folpet, Tebuconazole, Fenbuconazole, Propargite, Dimethoate, Heptachlor epoxide, Diazinon

Ingredients: Strawberry

Also, the following chart by Dr. Jockers reveals how toxicity leads to weight gain. So much of our soil, air, and environment are toxic. We cannot avoid it, so we must make a habit of detoxing/cleansing our bodies regularly. We have also included some ideas you can incorporate on a daily basis from an article published by *The Truth About Cancer*. You will find many items on the list very helpful and you can find out more by doing a little more research.

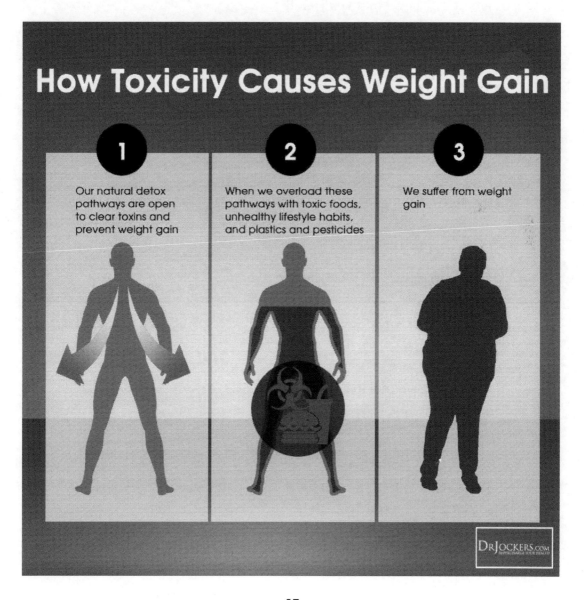

How Toxicity Causes Weight Gain

1 Our natural detox pathways are open to clear toxins and prevent weight gain

2 When we overload these pathways with toxic foods, unhealthy lifestyle habits, and plastics and pesticides

3 We suffer from weight gain

DrJockers.com

30 Ways to Naturally Detoxify Your Body Every Day
Source: Edited Version of Detox List from *The Truth About Cancer* (TTAC)

#1. Drink more purified water. It takes liquid to flush out those unwanted toxins. Try upping your hydration level today by taking your total weight, dividing it in half, and consuming that much in ounces of fresh, filtered, good-for-you water. You'll be amazed by how great you'll feel!

#2. Start your day with lemon water. Get the hydration habit going with 8 oz. before you eat or drink anything else. Use real lemon juice or, if you are on the go, simply add 1 drop of supplement-grade lemon essential oil to your water.

#3. Oil Pulling. Oil pulling is the process of swishing 1 tablespoon organic coconut oil around in your mouth for between 10 and 20 minutes. The chemical reaction between your saliva and the oil literally "pulls" bacterial toxins out from the deepest crevices in your whole oral cavity. According to Dr. F. Karach, oil pulling can also strengthen the stomach, heart, liver, lungs, and reproductive organs. Give it a try – and don't forget to spit it out afterwards into the garbage can so you don't clog your sink drain.

#4. Tongue Scraping. Besides oil pulling, another effective way to target the oral cavity for detoxification is through the Ayurvedic practice of "tongue scraping." According to Sheila Patel, MD, medical director at the Chopra Center, "Scraping the tongue daily removes any build-up on the tongue, which, if left untreated, …may house a significant number of bacteria." Tongue scraping requires an inexpensive tool that can be purchased at most pharmacies. Stainless steel works well, says Patel. The tongue should be scraped very gently from back to front 7 to 14 times.

#5. Eat more organic green leafy veggies. Kale, spinach, parsley, cilantro, and celery… all these greens are your friends. They contain vital nutrients, plenty of fiber, and chlorella, which helps to cleanse the blood. Try them in a smoothie or very lightly sautéed in coconut oil if eating them raw is not for you.

#6. Add some Prebiotics. The gut is the first line when it comes to nutrient absorption, and prebiotics are the "food" of healthy gut bacteria. Most health food stores now have pre-made, probiotic rich raw sauerkraut and kimchi. Look for it in the refrigerated aisle and add it to your lunch today!

#7. Try some chlorophyll. Another great addition to your diet can be chlorophyll in tablet or liquid form. Chlorophyll is the green pigment found in plants and algae. Chlorophyll can increase red blood cells and bind with toxins and heavy metals, sending them on their way and out of your body.

#8. Consider gentle detoxifying teas. Add some dandelion, turmeric, or Holy Basil tea to your evening routine, or try lemon tea for a mid-afternoon pick-me-up. Chia, milk thistle, garlic, and spirulina are all great natural detoxifiers and heavy metal chelators as well.

#9. "Unplug" during a meal. Take a media break while you eat. This is just a good habit to get in for proper digestion. While you eat your lunch or as you sit down with your family for dinner, instead of focusing on who is texting you or what is playing on TV, why not focus on what is going on around you or with each other? Chew your food slowly as well – chewing is the first stage of digestion.

#10. Media detox. Why not extend your non-media mealtime to a whole day "unplugged?" Abstain from watching the news and other sensationalized or violent television and movies. Opt to read a book, go for a walk, listen to some music, or do a craft instead. At the end of the day, write down how you felt before and after your "media detox."

#11. Use an essential oil. Essential oils can be a great adjunct to your detoxing goals. Experiment with peppermint to refresh the mind, oregano to help with viruses and bacteria, frankincense which has many benefits, etc.

#12. Bentonite clay, anyone? Clay is a powerful anti-bacterial. It can help get rid of viruses such as E. coli, MRSA, and Staphylococcus. Plus, it is great for heavy metal detox as well. Try mixing a tiny amount of pesticide-free bentonite clay powder in an 8-oz. glass of water. If you decide to continue using bentonite clay more often, start slowly and work your way up to a teaspoon or more.

#13. Play out your stress. Take a detox from the mundane and dive into your creativity! Spend at least an hour engaging in a healthy creative activity, allowing all concepts of time to go out the window. Get lost in the play of painting, dancing, writing, doodling, needlepoint, being in nature, or whatever brings you joy.

#14. Breathe more. Pay attention to your breath. Does your breathing become shallow when you are stressed or upset? Decide to take a deep breath instead. Deep breathing can help cleanse the respiratory system and oxygenate the blood.

#15. Try Meditation. Meditation not only calms the mind, it also helps relax those stress responses that are pumping too much cortisol into your body, creating inflammation and toxic build-up. Start with even 5 minutes and simply focus on your breath as you close your eyes, meditate on scripture, and create a "happy place" in your mind that creates peace.

#16. Do some aerobic exercise. Get moving! Aerobic exercise pumps life-giving oxygen and feel-good hormones into your body. But did you also know that, according to researchers at the Swedish Karolinska Institute, during a workout, the muscles act like the liver and produce an enzyme that clears out depression-causing chemicals?

#17. Stretch and release. Stretching not only keeps muscles and joints flexible, it can also lower inflammation and "fight or flight" responses that can lead to chronic disease. A 2009 study of women with breast cancer found that those who underwent a 75-minute restorative stretching class for 10 weeks had less instances of depression than those who did not. Stay motivated and detox from stress by doing a few stretches throughout the day.

#18. Hot and cold shower cycling. Now that you have worked up a sweat and stretched it all out, consider keeping the detoxing going as you step into the shower. Cold showers can lower stress and improve circulation. Hot showers, on the other hand, relieve tension and congestion and help you sleep better. Turn the shower temp to a little hotter than you would normally have it. Then alternate the temp to as cold as it will go for 30 seconds. Work up to alternating hot & cold intervals for 5-minutes.

#19. Spend time in nature. *Shinrin-yoku*, or "forest bathing," is a Japanese term for being in nature in order to gain the physical benefits it can offer. A 2010 review of 24 studies found that forest bathing kicks in parasympathetic nerve activity that can help heal and detoxify. Don't live near a forest? Try the beach, a park, an indoor greenhouse, or even a hotel courtyard.

#20. Get some sun today. Sunshine provides us with vital vitamin D, a truly "healing hormone" that has been linked to lower inflammation, lower blood pressure, improvements in muscle tone, improved brain function, and even cancer protection. Try 10-15 minutes of sun exposure without sunscreen (however, whenever you do need to use sunscreen, make sure you use a non-toxic brand). If you are in a part of the world that doesn't get much sun, consider investing in a "SAD lamp" or supplementing Vitamin D3.

#21. Make your home electro-pollution free. The National Institutes of Health recently released a report which proved the connection between close-range cell phone use and certain kinds of cancer. Cell phones are just one source of harmful EMFs, however. A few simple actions can turn your home into an "EMF-free zone." Make sure your bed is located as far away as possible from SMART meters. Turn off your Wi-Fi routers before you snooze so that EMFs do not disturb the quality sleep you need to detox and heal.

#22. Do a "purge" of your kitchen and bathroom. Take a look inside your kitchen and bathroom cabinets. Evaluate your sundry and beauty products as well as the items in your kitchen. The Environmental Working Group says that there are over 3,000 "stock chemical ingredients" that the perfume industry alone can choose from for their products, many of which have not been tested for safety. Switch out one commercial product at a time for an all-organic one and consider switching out at least one product a week until your home is truly toxin-free.

#23. Take a bath. "Hyperthermia," or using heat to heal, is a great detox modality. Your bathtub can be your own hyperthermia tool. Take a hot bath and release tension with some added Epsom or mineral salts and calming essential oils, like lavender. After getting out of the bath, wrap yourself in a blanket for a few minutes for some extra sweating power.

#24. Body brushing. Brushing your skin for detoxing? You bet! And right before a bath or shower is the best time to do it. Using a soft-bristle brush, gently start at your feet and arms and work your way towards your heart. Dry brushing is a core modality for Ayurvedic detoxification protocols because it stimulates the lymphatic system.

#25. Give an enema a try. Even though enemas are still fairly "taboo" in the United States, in other countries, such as India, they are as normal for routine health as brushing one's teeth. (You can read more about coffee enemas for cleansing the liver in other articles on TTAC.) A simple filtered or distilled water enema with a bit of aloe or lemon juice added, however, can be a soothing way of flushing the colon as well.

#26. Castor oil packs. Castor oil packs have been shown to improve the detoxification capacity of the liver, support reproductive organs, improve lymph flow, and reduce inflammation. Try using a castor oil pack along with a heat source on your abdomen for at least an hour.

#27. Foot massage. Relax and unwind by giving yourself a soothing foot massage. Reflexology is the Chinese practice of corresponding points on the foot with organs in the body. When you are massaging your feet, you are really loosening up the entire body. For a deep, reflexology massage, make a fist and use your knuckles to rub up and down with medium pressure on each point for up to one minute. Notice if there are any areas of soreness. Then check which organs these points correspond to on a reflexology chart.

#28. Connect with others. Connect with someone in your life that means a lot to you. Make a phone call or send a text just to say "hi." If no one is around, sit in a coffee shop or a park and strike up a conversation. If you don't see the link between social interaction and health, consider the well-known "Alameda County" study. It found that for every individual in the decades-long study, those with the fewest social ties were *three times more likely* to die over a 9-year period than those who had the most social ties. Importantly, this was regardless of pre-existing health conditions, socioeconomic status, smoking, alcohol consumption, obesity, race, sexual satisfaction, physical activity, and use of preventive health services. Wow!

#29. Take time for gratitude and appreciation. Detox from negative thinking by tuning in to the things, people, and situations in your life that you are most appreciative of. Have a job you love? Are your kids the bomb? Do you live in a great neighborhood? Are you grateful for all that you have learned about detoxing and your health? Celebrate all of this until it puts a smile on your face!

#30. Take time to pray. Last on this list, but certainly not least, take the time to simply *let go*. Say and practice the Serenity Prayer. Give things that are outside of your control – things that concern you and cause anxiety, worry, and stress – to GOD! (TTAC/detox)

BABY STEPS TO LIVING WELL – FIT 'n' FAITH

It takes 21-30 days to create a new habit. Therefore, as you consider the steps you need to take to become healthy and whole, it will be important to establish and make a choice that you can stay consistent with every 21-30 days. Lasting change takes time. If we try to change too many things all at once, it becomes overwhelming and seemingly impossible to sustain. One or two baby steps at a time, however, are manageable. How about this: even a 1% a day change of habit or mindset can lead to a complete transformation in your life in only 90 days! That's what we will pursue in the second half of this chapter. Welcome to the baby step journey.

PREPARING FOR THE JOURNEY

- **Pray** and then **Pray** some more! ☺

- Keep a food journal for at least 2 weeks to monitor your food choices. Also record emotions when you happen to eat more than you should, or when you eat specific things you know to be unhealthy. This journal helps us determine patterns of eating and types of food that may need to be eliminated for 90 days as your first baby step (trigger food to abstain from).

- Identify 1 or 2 main staples that you and your family have on a regular basis that could be the first change you make to eliminate toxins and increase nutrition – something you eat or drink a lot of on a regular basis (milk, cereal, meat, eggs, soda, cookies, etc.).

Baby Step 1

1. Replace those 1 or 2 items you identified above with the healthy counterpart (i.e., pasteurized milk to organic, almond, rice, coconut, cashew milk options; packaged cereals to fruit, Greek organic yogurt, steel cut oats with cinnamon, honey & walnuts; etc.).

2. Start thinking about investing in a blender, Magic Bullet, or Ninja, and start experimenting a bit with smoothies (the goal: at least 5 per week)

3. Possible STOPS: Stop Fast Food
                         Stop all Soda – regular and/or diet

4. DO: Eat an apple a day (preferably organic Granny Smith)

   DO: Soak all produce in vinegar (ACV or white distilled is fine) or a teaspoon or two of baking soda without aluminum, for 10 minutes, scrub & rinse before storing (removes pesticides, wax, and helps preserve)

5. Incorporate 1 "cheat day" per week – have anything you want but don't overdo it.

Baby Step 2 (Note: do not move "fully" into the next Baby Step until you have created a new habit)

1. Start drinking more water (goal over time: ½ your body weight in ounces). Purified water is best – start saving for a good in-home filter (might be a good way to spend that income tax refund check in the future!).

   Water makes up 70-75% of your total body weight. It helps you maintain body temperature and metabolize body fat, aids in digestion, lubricates and cushions organs, transports nutrients, and flushes toxins from our bodies. Add a squeeze of lemon for flavor on occasion or a drop of essential oil (be sure to use containers that are NOT plastic or at least Non-BPA – glass or stainless steel are best especially when using essential oils). Herbal teas also count for water intake, so experiment with some new flavors.

2. Meatless Mondays, Tuesdays, Wednesdays, Thursdays, or Fridays, any one or two days a week. Your body can only process 3-4 ounces of protein every 4-6 hours. When eating meat, estimate a serving size by clenching your fist. This is how much you should be eating. So...have a meatless dish once a week or more – give your body and grocery bill a break. An added boost would be to eat "clean" meat. No bottom feeder meats, and purchase grass fed beef, free range chickens/eggs, and NO shell fish – refer to healing foods shopping list by Dr. Axe in the Appendix.

3. Buying Organic – Choose your produce wisely. Stick to purchasing ONLY organic from the list below. All others can be non-organic but wash all properly (soak in vinegar: add ¼ - ½ cup to sink filled with water) for at least 10 minutes, then scrub and rinse well.

Buy Organic Only (below)

Apples	Sweet bell peppers	Celery
Peaches	Potatoes	Spinach
Nectarines	Hot peppers	Cucumbers
Strawberries/All Berries	Kale and Collard greens	Tomatoes
Grapes	Snap peas	

Baby Step 3

1. Cut your caffeine consumption to 1-2 cups in the morning. Caffeine dehydrates and leaches important minerals from our bones. Anytime we consume caffeine, we should always increase our water intake. If possible, switch to an organic coffee you can brew at home.
   Do you like creamer in your coffee? Switch to coconut or almond milk. Green tea is another alternative to getting a bit of caffeine and at the same time consuming a beverage that is high in anti-oxidants – try some of the flavored organic brands – they are wonderful.

2. Breakfast!!! Before you put coffee, tea, or food into your body, it is best to first start your day with water (lemon added would be even better). Having water before we eat helps our body to absorb nutrients from the food and/or smoothie we will eat that morning, and the lemon helps rebalance our digestive tract by making it alkaline. Eat Breakfast! – a green smoothie would be perfect (greens, fruit, protein powder, coconut oil).

3. Are you still eating an apple a day? Time to add more significant veggies that detox the body if you haven't already – beets and/or carrots. You can add them to a smoothie or have them raw or roasted. Beets bind toxins, heavy metals, and excess hormones that are dumped into the gut from the liver; beets will allow them to be passed out instead of being reabsorbed. Carrots bind toxins, bile acids, hormones, and heavy metals as well. Enjoy some of each every day or at least fit them in several times a week.

4. Rest, Eliminate Some Stress – Take time to evaluate your calendar, priorities, and goals to make some needed changes. Incorporate times of Sabbath rest. Get at least 7-9 hours of sleep each night. Do you have trouble sleeping? There are natural alternatives to sleeping pills: kava kava, melatonin, calcium with magnesium (calm), lavender oil, and aromatherapy are great options.

Baby Step 4

1. Eat "living" food (as much raw as possible). When eating cooked foods, be sure to take a quality digestive enzyme and take a probiotic every day. Add some nuts and seeds (<u>raw</u>: almonds, walnuts, cashews, pistachios, pumpkin seeds, sunflower seeds).

2. Change to healthy grains – quinoa; whole grain breads; Ezekiel bread (in the freezer section); use a whole, multi-grain, rice or quinoa pasta – better yet, spaghetti squash is wonderful.

3. Exercise – get moving and especially spend some time outside even in the winter months. We need 10-15 minutes a day of sun exposure to create the vitamin D necessary for health and mood.

   • Sweat! Our bodies store toxins in fat so...start finding ways to sweat! Check out some workouts from the library (books, DVDs) and start working on this a bit more. Take a class (Stretch & Strength/Praise Moves), start walking, or join a gym. If you want to purchase equipment, something that is very low cost and excellent for the lymphatic system and getting some sweat going is a rebounder (mini-trampoline). Keep in mind – the key to peak fat burning with any exercise is to be able to talk without being winded. Try some "surge" exercising (more on that in chapter 9).

4. Supplements & Such – Daily, begin taking:

   • a water soluble, whole food multi-vitamin
   • 5000 IU Vitamin D3 daily in the winter, 2000-3000 IU in the summer
   • Krill or Flaxseed Oil for Omega 3's
   • Pink Air-Dried sea salt
   • Apple Cider Vinegar – at least 1 Tbsp a day (preferably at night); take more if you can

Baby Step 5

1. Fresh Air! Our homes become stale and filled with toxins. Air out your home regularly even in the winter months. Turn down the thermostat and open the windows for five minutes every few weeks.

2. Whole body detox – do this quarterly. A good way to remember is to do so at the change of seasons. There are several kits on the market that you can get at the health food store or online. A couple of good brands are "Garden of Life" and "Enzymatic".

3. Sweeteners – Switch to: xylitol, stevia, raw organic honey, powdered monk fruit, dates, figs, pure maple syrup.

4. Oral Hygiene – Use Tom's with no fluoride or Spry (gum and mints too) or make your own:

   - coconut oil
   - baking soda (with no aluminum)
   - essential oils like peppermint, clove, thieves, etc.

   (Ratio: 2 parts coconut oil to 1 part baking soda with 10-15 drops of essential oils each – try using 2 different essential oils at a time).

5. Deodorants/soaps – find brands at the health food store or online that do not have all the added chemicals and aluminum that are cancer causing agents (ideas: Kiss My Face, Native, Schmidts).

Baby Step 6

1. What is your largest organ? Skin!!!! It absorbs 60% of what we put on it. Consider installing a carbon-block water filter on your shower head – the cost is minimal (around $45 for the initial purchase with replacement filters thereafter); the goal is to reduce our daily intake of toxins – especially the fluoride and chlorine.

2. Consider homeopathic remedies. For colds/flu (as soon as symptoms begin):

   - Apple cider vinegar
   - Elderberry
   - Echinacea
   - Umcka
   - Zinc
   - Oscillococcinum

   - 1000 mg. Vitamin C every 3-4 hrs
   - ACV with raw honey and cinnamon
   - Thieves and/or oregano essential oil
   - Essiac Tea (includes burdock root, slippery elm, sheep sorrel, Indian rhubarb root)

3. Cleaning products – check the ingredients of what you currently use. Begin changing to a healthier option from a health-conscious company, or use some of the easiest and cheapest non-toxic options available: baking soda, hydrogen peroxide, distilled white vinegar. For added antibacterial benefits for your cleaner, include a few drops of an essential oil (tea tree, lemon, orange, thieves, eucalyptus). Equal parts vinegar and water with a bit of hydrogen peroxide make a great all-purpose cleaner. Or water, hydrogen peroxide and a couple of drops of essential oil is great for cleaning spots on carpets – works great for pet stains too.

Note: Always keep in mind that at any point in time you feel overwhelmed and the step you are on becomes unmanageable, go back to the prior step and persevere until you are ready to move forward. The only caution here is you must move forward at some point to enjoy the kind of health and wholeness God desires for you and your family. The process outlined above could be spread out over the course of a year – it is attainable – stick to it, you will NOT regret it!!!

6

WEAPONS OF MASS DISTRACTION

Staying the Course

"Never confuse motion with action" – Benjamin Franklin

Modern living and technology have programmed us for distraction. We can be like the talking dogs in the cartoon movie *Up* when they're focused on one thing and then suddenly distracted: *"Oh look, squirrel!!"* They were always so easily sidetracked. ☺ We, too, can be diverted into the trivial in a split second. Movies and videos change scenes as quickly as every one to two seconds, and this doesn't help matters. This was not always the case. The information age has caused much distraction. We used to sip, as it were, from the fountain of knowledge, but now we drink information daily from a fire hose, and the numerous items on our "to do list" are like children screaming out to be chosen for the team: *Pick me! Pick me!*

The disappearance of margin has been creeping into your life without you even realizing it. Quantity, not quality, is the theme of the age we now live. We experienced a refreshing and living example of the opposite just a few years ago as we traveled to Africa on our first missions trip. As Lillian said, it was like going back in time: slow-paced living, meaningful conversations, slow enjoyable meals, and no clock watching. This is much closer to what we believe is useful and productive for wholeness of life, whether pursuing fitness or living out lives of faith. We suggest you give it a try – linger longer in conversation, find God's glory in the ordinary, and gain freedom from slavery to the clock. We understand this is very counter-cultural, and to do so may seem difficult after being controlled by the tyranny of the "treadmill of life" for so long. Staying instead of straying will produce peace and purpose, and you can be a great example of a balanced life to those you love.

Luci Swindoll shares a story that further illustrates this:

Several years ago I read a story that often comes to mind when I think about the wisdom of taking life slowly.

It seems that some African missionaries had hired a number of native workers to carry their supplies from one village to another. The missionaries, possessed of the American "push-rush-hurry" mentality, verbally prodded their native employees every day to go a little faster and a little farther than they had the day before. Finally, after three days of being pushed and hurried, the native workers sat down and refused to move.

"What in the world is the problem?" the American missionaries wanted to know. "We have been making excellent time. There's no need to stop here."

"It is not wise to go so rapidly," the spokesman for the native workers explained. "We have moved too fast yesterday. Now today we must stop and wait here for our souls to catch up with our bodies."

Don't you love that? "Wait here for our souls to catch up with our bodies." What a powerful philosophy.

Pausing for a moment here and there takes conscious effort, especially at first, but it will eventually become a habit, and the habit will turn into a way of life. In fact, it will most probably become a foundation stone in one's value system, because we simply cannot live fully or wisely without slowing down, without putting on the brakes, without awareness of each moment. ("Several Years Ago....")

Are you Staying or Straying? What's your squirrel (like the dogs' distractions from the movie *Up*)**?**

Spend a few moments thinking and praying through this question and write down what comes to mind: What are your current distractions that keep you from the goal God has in mind for your life?

It takes work to stay on course, so you need to throw daily counter punches at the mass distraction bully.

GOD'S WEAPONS OF MASS PROTECTION

Here are just a few samples of God's weapons of mass protection that you should have ready and available to use. Memorize them or keep them visible on a 3x5 card, screen saver, etc. Take the time right now to look up each of these passages and jot down a few words that stand out for you that are messages to cling to as God's protection.

Philippians 4:6 NIV
Isaiah 26:3 NLT
Jeremiah 29:13 NLT

Proverbs 4:25-27 NLT
Philippians 3:15-16 MSG

6 ESSENTIALS TO LIVING WELL (a Fit 'n' Faith lifestyle)

As we consider staying the course and pursuing our goal of wholeness, these essentials always need to be at the forefront of our mind – the essentials that will get us there.

- A Renewed Mind: Continue to re-frame your thinking and monitor self-talk
- Quality Nutrition: Increase organics, reduce processed foods
- Oxygen & Lean Muscle: Deep breathing and exercise
- Minimize Toxins & Detox: Detox quarterly with a whole-body cleanse
- Nerve Supply: See a chiropractor regularly, get a massage
- H_2O: Half your body weight in ounces of purified/filtered water

Focus on all the parts: Body, Soul, Spirit

PREPARING & PLANNING TO STAY THE COURSE (a few more helpful tools)

- Write down what you eat.
- Properly fuel your body. The following image provides a concept of what types of foods you can eat and the equivalent in calories of what will help you feel satisfied.

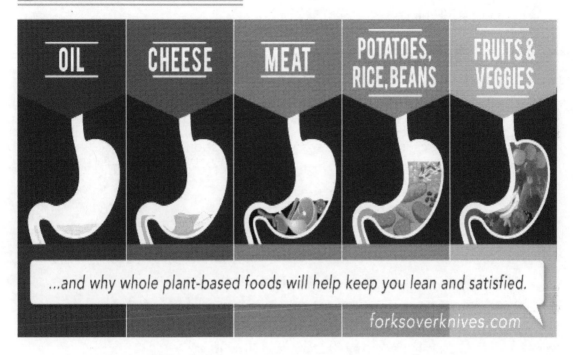

CALORIE DENSITY WHAT 500 CALORIES LOOK LIKE

| OIL | CHEESE | MEAT | POTATOES, RICE, BEANS | FRUITS & VEGGIES |

...and why whole plant-based foods will help keep you lean and satisfied.

forksoverknives.com

WHAT ABOUT FASTING – would it help?

Dr. Don Clum is a Chiropractor, a functional fitness expert, and a specialist in Advanced Metabolic Nutrition. He states:

There are many ways to fast and to get the powerful benefits of fasting, such as:

1. Juice fasting
2. Fat fasting
3. Fasting-mimicking diet
4. Pseudo fasting

5. Rotational fasting
6. Intermittent fasting
7. Water fasting
8. Block fasting

And probably a few more.

Dr. Clum goes on to share this Doctor/patient interaction:

Doctor: "Fasting causes your body to go into starvation mode!"

Me: No more than drinking water causes you to go into drowning mode.

Doctor: "Fasting lowers your metabolism!"

Me: No, it raises it when tested.

Doctor: "Fasting is too hard on the body!"

Me: No, when done right and following the proper progression, it is extremely easy on your body and healing.

Doctor: "You will get hypoglycemia (low blood sugar) if you fast!"

Me: No, you won't.

Doctor: "Your brain needs regular glucose to run itself!"

Me: It needs less than you think and your body can make all it needs without food.

I could go on and on.

NOTE: You can learn a lot about your health by fasting. How your body does over time without food is a great measure of how resilient and healthy it is. If you CAN'T skip even a single meal or snack, or even one day of eating without major issues, then yes, you do have major issues, but not due to the fasting.

Dr. Clum goes on to say:

The best way I have found to approach this is to make a long-term plan and build up to different levels of fasting. I have tried them all and last year did a full 30-day fast myself.

The fasting state is natural and works different metabolic, hormonal, and neurological pathways than the feeding state does. Most people need to train these pathways like one would to get in shape in the gym, with regular effort over time. But when done right, the "fitness" on the other side is amazing and worth it.

Quick tips from Dr. Clum:
1. One week before a fast, take all insoluble fiber out of your diet.
2. Start small and work your way up; as in, start with just eating 3 meals a day and no snacking.
3. Yes, you can drink water, coffee, tea or organic broth if it helps, in the beginning.
   Something is better than nothing and over time it gets easier and the experience better. Give it a shot, you will actually SAVE money by doing this; then invest that money into more advanced health efforts, whole foods, or programs.

By the way, skipping breakfast is NOT intermittent fasting. Deciding not to eat a meal, or even multiple meals, is a matter of meal timing variation and not really a true fast at all. Even skipping a full day is not traditionally considered fasting. Traditionally, intermittent fasting was considered a 3 day to 20 day fast multiple times over a year or more. True fasting was considered anything 21 days or more. Regardless of how fasting is defined, there is value in understanding it better.

Skipping a meal or even a day of eating is not abnormal. In some older cultures still in existence, periodically by choice, seasonal fasting is common and has been for centuries (partially due to food scarcity). There is absolutely nothing wrong, unhealthy, or problematic about not eating for what we would now consider long periods of time.

In fact, the fasting physiology is powerfully health-promoting and healing. Think of animals in nature or your experience when you have had the flu—you innately lose your appetite when ill. Why would that be? We may not know, but the body knows what it is doing and was designed to do (by God of course).

During fasting, our body cleans house, literally. Our body recycles old damaged, poorly functioning cells, pumps healing hormones, trims dangerous fat out of our muscles and organs, de-frags our brain, and reboots the immune system. It is truly amazing! (We are fearfully and wonderfully made.)

Intermittent Fasting is a great early to mid-program practice in a rotational fasting or health recovery protocol to gear up to bigger fasting efforts. It is also great to boost health efforts, weight loss, and maintenance.

– Edited version of Dr. Don's Facebook post Feb, 2018.

Here are a few recommendations to try from Dr. Axe & Jordan Rubin:
Pick one of the following as your Eating Window:

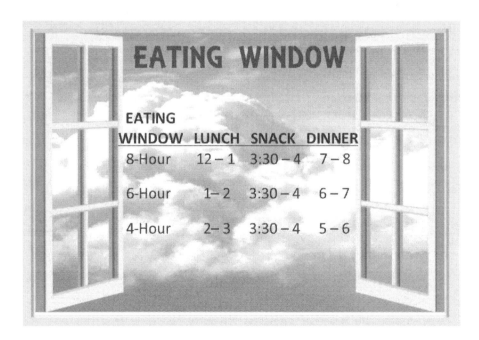

EATING WINDOW

EATING WINDOW	LUNCH	SNACK	DINNER
8-Hour	12 – 1	3:30 – 4	7 – 8
6-Hour	1– 2	3:30 – 4	6 – 7
4-Hour	2– 3	3:30 – 4	5 – 6

All of the above are times for eating solid food. The good news is that you can enjoy satisfying beverages throughout the day.

Start with 2 days a week, then move to 3, and you are off to the races. There are other options in the charts that follow (benefits and types).

As part of a recent physical and spiritual challenge, we are doing a 30-Day progressive fast. Feel free to give this one a try or another and see how it goes!

30-Day Progressive Fast

Week #1 – Pick 2 Days and fast as follows:

Practice the 8-Hour Eating Window: 12 – 1 Lunch,   3:30 – 4 Snack,   7 – 8 Dinner

Week #2 – (2 Days):

Practice the 6-Hour Eating Window: 1 – 2 Lunch,   3:30 – 4 Snack,   6 – 7 Dinner

Week #3 – (2 Days):

Practice the 4-Hour Eating Window: 2 – 3 Lunch,   3:30 – 4 Snack,   5 – 6 Dinner

You can either choose to do 2 days consecutively or skip a day or two in between.
Note: The snack allowance is "if needed"; skip it if you can.

Final Week – A full day (or two) fast with liquids only.

Benefits of
FASTING

1 BOOSTS WEIGHT LOSS

A 2015 study found that alternate day fasting trimmed body weight by up to 7 percent and slashed body fat by up to 12 pounds. (1)

2 PROMOTES SECRETION OF HUMAN GROWTH HORMONE

Naturally produced by the body, HGH is used to treat obesity and help build muscle mass, important for burning fat.

3 HELPS ATHLETES

Fasting has been found to have positive effects on body mass as well as other health markers in professional athletes.

4 NORMALIZES INSULIN SENSITIVITY

A World Journal of Diabetes study found that intermittent fasting in adults with type-2 diabetes improved key markers for those individuals, including their body weight and glucose levels. (2)

5 NORMALIZES GHRELIN LEVELS

Known as the hunger hormone, ghrelin levels can stabilize with fasting (unlike with dieting).

6 LOWERS TRIGLYCERIDE LEVELS

Intermittent fasting lowers those bad cholesterol levels, decreasing triglycerides in the process. (3)

7 MAY SLOW DOWN THE AGING PROCESS

While not yet proven in humans, early studies in rats seem to link intermittent fasting with increased longevity. (4)

(1) https://www.ncbi.nlm.nih.gov/pubmed/26374764
(2) https://www.ncbi.nlm.nih.gov/pmc/articles/PMC5394735/
(3) https://www.ncbi.nlm.nih.gov/pubmed/19793855
(4) https://www.ncbi.nlm.nih.gov/pubmed/21021020

Dr. Axe

Types of
FASTING

WHAT IS FASTING?
Abstaining from food and drink from a specific period of time

Spiritual fasting is a part of many religions. Increasingly, it's become popular as part of health regimens to detox, lose weight, etc.

TYPES OF FASTS

INTERMITTENT FASTING

"Cyclic fasting" range from 14–18 hours

TIME-RESTRICTED EATING

Abstain from food for anywhere between 12–16 hours

16/8 FASTING

Like time-restricted eating, fasting for 16 hours a day and then eat the other 8

ALTERNATE DAY FASTING

Severely restricting the amount of calories you eat during fasting days (about 25% of your normal intake), then eating to your stomach's content on non-fasting days

THE 5:2 DIET

Eat normally for 5 days of the week, then eat only 500–600 calories on each of the other 2 days

THE WARRIOR DIET

Stick to fruits and veggies during the day, then eat a well-rounded, larger meal in the evenings

THE DANIEL FAST

Based off of Daniel's experiences in the Bible's Book of Daniel, this 21-day fast features vegetables, fruits and other healthy whole foods prominently while meat, dairy, grains (unless they're sprouted ancient grains) and drinks like coffee, alcohol and juice are avoided

Dr. Axe

WHAT ABOUT GUT HEALTH?

Much of what we have shared in this chapter can help you with gut health. It is said that the gut is the second brain, and most people do not realize that 70-80% of the immune system lies in the intestinal tract/gut.

Dr. David Brownstein, M.D. is a board-certified family physician and one of the nation's foremost practitioners of holistic medicine, and the Medical Director of the Center for Holistic Medicine in West Bloomfield, Michigan. According to Dr. Brownstein, millions of people suffer silently from a serious health problem related to a lack of gut health or parasite invasions. Sadly, most don't even know it.

According to an article written by Dr. Brownstein:

The problem starts out mildly enough — barely even noticeable. The symptoms may be commonplace or may not seem to be related to the true cause.

You belch a lot after dinner. Or worse, pass a little wind at an unfortunate moment. No big deal, happens to everybody.

Your acne flares up. So what? Happens at any age.

You're a little more tired than usual. Well, aren't we all?

That nasty heartburn and acid reflux happen more frequently. Your stomach hurts. Your joints ache. Pollen is wreaking havoc on your sinuses.

Sound familiar? Most are shocked when they discover they're suffering from a very common digestive ailment. Yet most mainstream doctors have never heard of it.

It may be why it's considered America's #1 undiagnosed health condition. It's called Leaky Gut Syndrome (LGS).

How "Leaky Gut" Affects You

Modern life is tough on your digestive system. Stress, environmental toxins, bacteria, and processed food can really take a toll on your gastrointestinal (GI) tract. Even the medications your doctor gives you can irritate your gut.

All of that irritation can cause tiny pinpricks in the delicate lining of your small intestine. As a result, undigested food, bacteria, and toxins can leak through the intestinal wall and enter your bloodstream. This can damage your immune system and your health.

Your gut is designed to absorb the vitamins, minerals, and nutrients you eat to nourish the rest of your body and give you energy. And your gut also gets rid of the bad things that hurt your body.

But with a leaky gut, nutrient absorption is compromised — and the bad things, like bacteria and toxins, escape the GI tract and enter your bloodstream.

In addition to painful digestive distress, a leaky gut also causes widespread inflammation. This inflammation can lead to your body's immune system attacking the body itself...and may be the root cause of many chronic illnesses today.

On the next page is a small test you can take to see if you might possibly have issues with the gut. Most of us do in varied degrees which is why we have been encouraging you to detox, eat clean, and practice fasting and cleansing on a regular basis. The first step in improving our gut is removing the things that are damaging it such as: artificial sweeteners, sugar, non-organic produce, GMOs (genetically modified food sources that are notorious for high levels of glyphosate), overly sterilized environments and antibiotics (destroy both good and bad bacteria). All of these contribute to an overgrowth of unwanted bacteria that can lead to sugar cravings, brain fog, increased risk of obesity, and more.

If you have serious gut issues, we recommend an assessment be done with a local naturopathic doctor such as Dr. Brownstein, or if you are suspect of issues with parasites, you need to have a team of professionals working with you to get these serious issues treated. After you have addressed the basics, like removing the healthy bacteria destroyers and getting lots of healthy fiber to feed your good bacteria, it will be helpful to introduce fermented vegetables or a high-quality probiotic supplement. In fact, we recommend either or both to be introduced in everyone's food plan daily regardless of your current situation, but for those who have been diagnosed or need to get an assessment because of serious symptoms, we recommend the cleansing protocol they discuss with you be done first (there is a variety including certain types of fasts, essential oil protocols that are followed for a period of time, etc.). Feel free to check the web sites of other professionals listed on the Resources page for further information.

The Leaky Gut Quiz

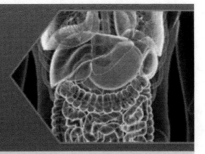

You may have a leaky gut if you suffer from:

	Yes	No
Bloating after you eat	☐	☐
Food allergies	☐	☐
Constipation/diarrhea	☐	☐
Acid reflux	☐	☐
Heartburn	☐	☐
Nausea	☐	☐
Dull stomach ache	☐	☐
Difficulty losing weight	☐	☐

Heal Your Leaky Gut.

7

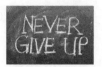

TESTIMONIES & MESS-TIMONIES

Perseverance not Perfection!

OUR STORIES

Following are a few stories from individuals who have gone through the 30-Day Jumpstart Lifestyle Change Program.

TARA:
I am not a morning person by any means. I always have trouble getting out of bed. I always set an alarm a half hour early and then snooze it and go back to sleep. Well I've been so awake since starting the challenge that I'm going to have to set my alarm for when I actually need to be up so I can enjoy that extra half hour of sleep instead of lying in bed wide awake. LOL

DENISE:

Here's an interesting observation. I fell asleep with socks on and once removed there was just a tiny indentation around my ankles. In the past it would have been very obvious I had socks on. Guess there's no fluid retention going on over here.

PAM & RON:

We are half way through and doing great! No more insulin shots for Ron, pants getting baggy, and feeling great!!! At the end of the 30: Ron just went to the doctor; he lost 20 pounds and his a1c was 7.1 last visit. This visit 6.0. The doctor is taking him off another medication. We cannot thank you enough for what you do.

NANCY:

To quote James Brown, "I feel good." Better than I thought I would. This has been a great journey for me. It was easier than I thought for a couple of reasons. My carb cravings were extinguished with tools from my recovery toolbox – another reason to thank God. But most importantly, I have been traveling a road of obedience and this was a side trip I needed to take. I grew closer to God during this time as I allowed Him to enter a new room in my life. At times it was as if I was a young child asking my parents "What do you want me to buy at the grocery store?" and "What should I have for dinner tonight?" And because of this attitude of heart, my eating became a more spiritual event rather than a physical or emotional one. I feel a much higher level of gratitude for all that He gives me on a daily basis. And, by bringing Him with me, our relationship has grown exponentially. I feel the moments of craving or the desire to run to food when my emotions are in upheaval, but I am trying to be dependent on Him for what I really need which, of course, is more of Him. My plan is to continue this "food boot camp" beyond the 30 days, adding a few things (chocolate and salmon perhaps) with His permission of course, and with some clear rules for their use. I will look to Lillian for some help. Thank you so much, Lillian, for your knowledge, support, and prayers.

JIM & NICOLE:

My wife and I finished our 30 days yesterday. We weighed in this morning and were very pleased with the results. I lost 16# and 4 inches off my waist. My wife lost 14# and 3 inches. When we started I was just hoping to lose 10#; never expected these results. If you stick to the plan it works!!

M:

Q1: What were the physical benefits you received from doing the 30?

Each time I did the challenge (I'm on my 3rd time) I lost weight & inches, which is good...but the more important change for me physically was that my blood sugar levels showed a drastic improvement. I found that I am actually able to keep them under much tighter control than previously, which is very important as I have diabetes.

Q2: Mental benefits?

I became much better at planning and preparing for my meals. I felt like I was controlling food, my use of it, rather than letting it control me!

Q3: Spiritual benefits?

The spiritual results of following this challenge were tremendous for me. I have misused and abused this temple God has given me for years, no – decades. Now that I am finally making a concentrated effort to treat my temple with the respect it...He...deserves, I feel that He is pleased with me. In addition, I believe that it is also pleasing to Him that I am going to Him when I am upset about something rather than going to food. I feel so much closer to Him than ever before!

ELIZABETH:

I slept on the floor last night with our grandkids – I could not believe that I slept there all night! The last time they slept over was a few months ago, and I didn't last more than ½ hour – I was stiff and sore and couldn't get comfortable. It must be the supplements – the oils? – my joints, my back, my neck – all of them were fine! Amazing! And I lost 27 pounds!

DENISE:

Q1: Were there parts of the program that were difficult for you and how did you overcome them?

The most difficult part of the program for me was twofold: 1) I genuinely love all kinds of foods that are not good for me – I love to eat, and 2) I am an emotional eater. I thought hunger was going to be a huge issue the first time I did the program, but I found that wasn't the case. My appetite/desires were the real problem. I had to rely strongly on God to help me through my emotions and temptations. There is no way I could have done this without a lot of prayers, both my own and those of my support group.

Oh...I guess there was another part that was difficult. I'm a busy person (who isn't?) who doesn't really enjoy cooking. It is so much easier to eat out than to prepare my own food. Getting through this issue took a whole lot of planning and discipline. It wasn't easy, especially in the beginning, but the more I did it, the more it became a way of life...a good one!

Q2: What words of encouragement do you have for those considering the program?

You CAN do this! I really never thought I could and I fought hard against even trying, but when I finally committed to it, body, soul, and spirit, God got me through it. With the help of God and a good support system, you can too!

DEB:

Before I started the 30-Day Challenge, I had already been a participant in the Health & Wellness classes LifeCare offers and I'd learned a lot of things that helped me to make several positive changes (baby steps) towards improving my health. I was drinking more water, gave up all soda pop and alcohol. I had reduced the amount of processed foods in my diet and added more fruits, vegetables, and lean proteins. I was seeing improvements in my health, but I knew there was still room for improvement.

When I heard about the opportunity to do the 30-Day Challenge through LifeCare, I have to admit I was apprehensive at first because I wasn't sure I would be able to do something as strict as what this program seemed to be, but I really believed God was leading me to this. I've learned through the years that oftentimes when I've felt the Holy Spirit nudging me towards something that I feel incapable of doing, that is exactly the time that He's ordained for me and will equip me as I look to His strength and not my own. So I committed to the program, believing God was encouraging me to take further steps toward greater health.

The support and encouragement of the group during the 30-Day Challenge along with the leadership tips, recipes, and cooking classes were all tremendously helpful, along with the weekly assignments. I used the assignments to journal my thoughts and feelings as I went through the process, which really helped make it clear to me that God was truly directing me to a "Lifestyle Change" (not just another diet or eating program) and that surrendering this area of my life to Him was an act of worship, just as important as anything else I've given over to Him. I had read the following verse many times before but it really came alive to me in a new way during the challenge. Romans 12:1, "Therefore, I urge you, brothers, in view of God's mercy, to offer your bodies as living sacrifices, holy and pleasing to God – this is your spiritual act of worship."

At the end of the 30-Day Challenge I had lost 14 lbs and was feeling so much better that I decided to continue on for another 10 days on my own. I was sleeping better and had such a sense of peace and calm along with greater clarity, like a fog was lifted. I even had co-workers comment on how peaceful I seemed and wanted to know what I was doing for my skin! My sinuses were clearer and digestion improved. I had less pain and more flexibility and movement in my joints. Once I completed the extra 10 days, I had lost a total of 21 lbs and was feeling great!

I'm very grateful for God's providence in leading me to LifeCare! I've learned so much more about health and nutrition than I ever knew before, both through the Health & Wellness classes they offer and the 30-Day Challenge LifeCare has put together. If you decide to take this journey yourself, I can say with full confidence you will be very glad you did!

DONNA:

Q1: How did I benefit?

> I lost 16 lbs, 17 inches, bloated feeling is gone, more energy, less mood swings, better skin, nails and hair, lab work: total cholesterol 244 – down to 185, HDL 74 – down to 66, LDL 160 – down to 110, my triglyceride result was 43.

I learned how to deny myself; think things through before just doing it. I learned how to go to God more than food. I am happy to know I could do this and make the needed changes so I didn't have to go on medication. My food choices have changed so much and I am surprised how little most of us know about the truth. I would encourage anyone to do this. It opened my eyes in many ways. I would remind you to commit all the way; know it is only 30 days, and experience changes you could not imagine. It will break chains and set you free of the lies you believe. Preparation will be important for you, and keep remembering permanent change is a process. I am looking forward to so much more learning and growing.

8

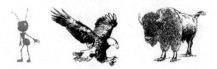

JOIN THE ANT, THE EAGLE, THE BUFFALO, AND *US!*

(The freedom of a "Fit 'n' Faith" lifestyle)

THE ANT

(Proverbs 6:6-8)—Ants provide plentifully against the time of famine. They never hinder but always assist one another in their work, and they can take on things that are too much for just one to handle. They take what is needed and vital to survive to places that the rain cannot reach. How do they make it through the winter? It's simple, they store in the summer when conditions are favorable. We should certainly know and apply this as it relates to God's temple (the body) and appreciate the fact that there are eternal investments at hand. With both our faith and our body, we need to be thinking ahead. If we're lax (and become sluggards, as the Bible defines it) and wait to start doing something about our health, the "winter season" comes and we can't maintain health or prevent spiritual or physical sickness.

The Cost and the COST (Prevention vs. Disease)

Nutrition, exercise, proper sleep, and daily Bible study are all prevention disciplines. Drawing near to God and doing what it takes to feel great are costly, but what is the cost of the alternative? Have you ever priced out a heart operation or cancer treatment and compared that to the "too expensive" health food? That's like comparing apples to hand grenades. I think I'll take the apples, thank you. Counting the cost now will save you much later.

Even the common cold or flu doesn't just happen. Over time, your immune system breaks down, and then "all of a sudden" you're sick. This process takes a while, but it happens in little bits and pieces.

No matter what your condition is now, your mind and body can be renewed by filling your "barns." Bible study, prayer, exercise, nutrition, etc. will make you the "ant" that can thrive in any "winter" conditions.

THE BUFFALO

So, let's say that you've done all that you can do and something still happens (as is life in this fallen world). Normally, we try to outrun the storms of life, but let's face it, you can't outrun them, can you? They *will* catch up to you, sooner or later. If you wait until later, you will have less fighting power and spend more time in the storm. Buffalo, unlike cattle and most other animals, face and move into storms that threaten. Buffalo charge into the storm, normally in a group, minimizing the time they spend in it. It's a powerful image to think of a herd of buffalo pushing forward in the face of a blizzard in the middle of Colorado, isn't it? Face the storms with all the strength, wisdom, knowledge, and faith you can.

THE EAGLE

(Excerpt from an article by columnist Solomon Benard July 21, 2009)

1. The eagle flies at altitudes far higher than any other bird. *You can rise above the norm and the storm.*

2. The eagle has amazingly strong vision. While in the air, it can see objects five kilometers away. *Keep your vision sharp and you will see the opportunities God has waiting for you.*

3. The eagle eats fresh prey. Whatever is stale or dead it won't touch. *Do away with dead things in your life.*

4. The eagle gets excited in the midst of a storm. It thrives in the storm and welcomes the gathering clouds. *We can thrive too!*

5. The eagle prepares for training. Male and female eagles take baby eagles to mountain tops at very high altitudes to prepare them to fly. The initial free fall is frightening, but the mother eagle comes to the rescue again and again until the baby eagle can fly alone at a high altitude. *Take faith risks – go ahead and jump – God will give you wings to fly or come to the rescue.*

Nature can teach us so much about the right way to live. My (Mike) primary pathway to God is in nature. I absolutely love being outside. Although I love our home, I don't sit well inside for long. Creation is so amazing and so are the creatures. Watching animals always makes me look at how I'm living my own life. Squirrels gather nuts, climb trees, etc. Bees build hives, make honey, etc. Birds nest and…. You get the point. Animals are doing exactly what God designed them to do—well…except mosquitoes. Why did God create them again? God designed us to worship Him, have relationship with Him as His precious children, and steward what He has graciously given us. Do you think it gives God glory to not care for the most precious gift He created, which is YOU?

We love to see elderly people holding hands and smiling at each other. How do you think they kept the spark of love and romance so long? By seeing marriage as a gift, and not neglecting to take care of that gift. Nurture and neglect both have lasting effects or consequences.

Dr. You and First Responders

First responders are the first ones on the scene of disasters to bring the necessary aid and supplies to save lives. They don't waste time; they can't second guess. They know what to do. Why? They've been trained for exactly this scenario. We must become our own doctor and first responder. We are not against doctors/medicine at all and would never downplay the need and vital importance of doctors, but when we neglect education in health, the doctors become the default to quick and easy relief (shots, pills, etc.).

God put his own "doctors" on earth that don't require insurance or appointments. Make a prevention appointment ASAP with Dr. Herb, Dr. Sun, and Dr. Plant to name a few.

There is no need to fear. Popular pharmacies/drug stores feed on the false fear factor of all the illnesses you're supposed to get every year. Get YOUR flu shot, shingles shot, etc. They give no explanation of what's in these shots or the effectiveness and risks. This is deception and what we call white-collar crime. Drug companies do their own research and publish their own papers on the safety and efficacy of the drugs they recommend. Every other TV commercial will tell you very slowly how great the drug is for whatever ails you, and then very quickly tell you the "possible" deadly side effects while still showing the smiling faces on the screen. Do you really need to face a stroke or heart attack to relieve your asthma?

In case an emergency happens, here are some basic first responders to common setbacks like the flu, headaches, insomnia, allergies, etc. (there are a few other ideas throughout the book).

- Vitamin D3 – builds up the immune system
- Essential Oils (See Chart in the Appendix)
- Curcumin/Turmeric – pain/inflammation, disease prevention
- Elderberry syrup with Echinacea – colds/flu symptoms
- Melatonin, Calm (magnesium & calcium combo), Valerian Root – sleep, also helps with stress and anxiety

US

Although far from perfect, we try to be lifelong learners, be good stewards, find mentors, learn from others' mistakes (and our own), create a new testimony, and deepen our faith. We are two sojourners who are passionate about Jesus, the gifts He's given, and helping people find the narrow path He's called us to, now and into eternity. Remember there is a narrow road to abundant life, and few truly find it.

The enemy of your body and soul has a powerful community that's out to destroy you and your life, so we need a community too! – Ants, buffalo, and eagles, we are!! Let's UNITE!!!

Preparing, facing, rising, joining – these are all critical to victory in the Fit 'n' Faith journey to wholeness.

We're all in this together. You can join the Fit 'n' Faith community by contacting us.

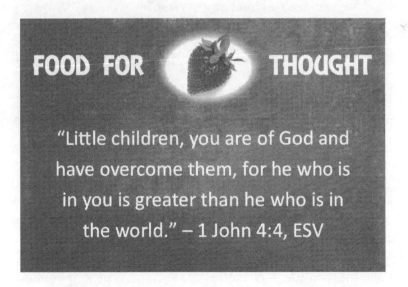

FOOD FOR THOUGHT

"Little children, you are of God and have overcome them, for he who is in you is greater than he who is in the world." – 1 John 4:4, ESV

You asked for it – You got it!

<u>**A PEEK INTO THE LIFE OF LILLIAN**</u>

I am pretty sure that many of you reading this book have gotten to a point when you say, "How in the world can I do all of this? How can I schedule it all in? It sounds impossible." At different points in time, I felt and thought the same thing. However, I have come to realize that if we all consider our current stage in life, the time we "REALLY" have to invest in lifestyle changes, we can begin our journey and make tremendous strides in no time with support and prayer. I had several people come to me over the years asking me what my schedule looks like as it relates to what I am teaching them and how can they make adjustments. Following is a brief synopsis of how I have been managing my changes over the last few years – a glimpse of my life – a glimpse of my schedule and how I have determined to manage a healthy lifestyle.

The night before, I prepare for the next day... What?

Prepare room temperature water in a glass bottle with 2-3 drops of lemon oil and leave by my coffee pot for the days I am not oil pulling. If it is an oil pulling day, I will leave my coconut oil out on the kitchen counter so it is easily accessible.

Smoothie prep: Most nights I prepare the majority of my smoothie for the next morning leaving out the coconut oil, flax and the protein powder since they have a tendency to stick to the sides or not blend well if I put them in the night before. I will put filtered water, veggies and fruits in so it is about half done and put it in the fridge in my magic bullet container.

Good Morning! Rise & Shine between 7 - 7:30am (weekdays)

I come downstairs and go directly to the kitchen counter and put 1tsp-1Tbsp of coconut oil in my mouth on the way to the bathroom if it is an "oil pulling day" (typically once a week is about all I do unless I am having dental problems). Otherwise, I stand at the counter and drink some of my lemon water before pouring my coffee and heading to the bathroom to get ready for the day while sipping my organic black brewed coffee.

After finishing up in the bathroom I head back to the kitchen to prepare my lunch/dinner bag for the day, and then I will take a few moments in my office to read, pray, check my calendar, check the weather for the day, etc.

Food Prep

I usually fill at least 3 containers (glass bottles) with filtered water, finish making my smoothie (to drink around 10 or 11am—I take my vitamins at that time too), and some of what I typically pack for the day would be any combination of:

- quinoa salad
- protein bars
- 1-2 pieces of fruit
- celery and organic peanut butter, almond butter or hummus or guacamole
- a nut mix I make with sunflower seeds, pumpkin seeds, almonds, cashews, etc.
- leftover soup
- a leafy green salad with a homemade dressing that has apple cider vinegar in it
- guacamole or hummus with veggies or healthy sprouted grain chips for dipping

If I need to bring something for a dinner snack because I am working late,
I add more to my lunch bag to hold me over and then have another small snack when I get home depending on the time. If I am really hungry and it is late, I will still eat something; I just try to make it light and no carbs. Sometimes I will have some of my:

- homemade fermented pickles
- pickled beets
- more veggies
- stuffed large olives

Big Cooking Days

Typically, I have 2-3 days that I cook large quantities of what can be frozen and/or eaten as leftovers. I make **quinoa** every week and add it into **stir fry, homemade vegan**

97

chili and even **soup,** or I use **brown or black rice**. Soups are great to make and they save you a ton of money – bean soups, veggie, etc.

Chili (2 or 3 bean like pinto, kidney, black) is always great with or without quinoa, or we make some sort of **Mexican bowl**. Another great dish if you like Mexican is **bean burritos** made with **refried lentils, pintos, or black beans** and **vegan cheese** (recipe is in the book). I will also make side dishes that last like:

- chick pea salad
- lentil or quinoa pasta salad
- quinoa salad
- all veggie salad with or without lettuce
- a spinach salad (listed in the recipe section)

Dinner Times

If I am still at work, Mike can enjoy the leftovers and any fresh produce we have. Other days, we will cook together and make **spaghetti squash with marinara** and whatever I have on hand to add, sprinkled with a **vegan cheese** or **nutritional yeast**. We will also use **quinoa or brown rice pasta**. Side dishes like a **quinoa and kale combination** is always good with **garlic**. We will make a healthy version of **pizza** for the days we need to be quick, or we will have a **black bean burger, quinoa/kale burger,** or **veggie burger on Ezekiel bread or Angelic bread or without bread** at all. **Boiled organic potatoes** are a hit in our household with a **pure organic butter** or **ghee**. We enjoy many fresh and/or frozen **organic veggies** such as:

- asparagus
- Brussels sprouts
- non-GMO corn (only occasionally)
- okra
- green beans

...all spiced up and roasted or steamed, then add a dab of butter on occasion and sea salt, pepper, and any other spices we have on hand.

Every Day

- I pray and get some truth in my mind whether it is while driving, sitting still, between clients, or in my bed at night reading the Word and multiple books (yes, at the same time – no worries, I do finish them eventually), and I talk to God all day long.

- I put an alarm on my Google Calendar to remind me to stretch 5-15 minutes every day and do a full 30-60 minute workout 3 days a week: cardio (e.g., biking outside when weather permits, walking, surge workout), stretch and weights or bands for strength training.

Shopping and Such

We do a very large, stock up on everything, shopping day once a month from Costco. Then weekly, we will run out and pick up odds and ends that we need from various markets, health food stores, and grocery stores that sell quality food items.

9

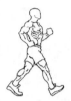

I LOVE YOU. I HATE YOU.
I NEED YOU!

"Exercise is wonderful," said Louis. "I could sit and watch it all day." – Larry Niven

"My grandmother started walking five miles a day when she was sixty. She's ninety-seven, and we don't know where she is now." (*edited version*) – Ellen DeGeneres

DANGER, QUILLS AHEAD!

I (Mike) once heard exercise likened to kissing a porcupine. They're cute, but you don't want to get close enough for a kiss because it could be very painful. How true this is about exercise. We know it's good and helpful to us for the long term, but we don't want to embrace it because of the possible pain and discomfort it may cause.

Exercise is God's anti-depressant and penicillin prescription wrapped into one. Yes, it may hurt for a bit when the pill goes down or the needle goes in, but oh how profitable it is when the results play out over days and years.

This chapter is a very condensed version about what we teach concerning exercise – the types and their benefits. We want to touch on this very important root that is a stabilizer of a strong and sturdy tree of whole, healthy living.

THE TV SHOW THAT COULD COST YOU YOUR LIFE

American *Idle* is a show that you don't want to be the star of. Idleness is costing the workplace millions of dollars and profiting doctors and pharmacists billions and billions. Multiple studies show that sitting is considered the new smoking. Being inactive can break your bank physically and financially. Let's face it, technology is making it easier to push, press, click, and wait for results, whether it be in the mind or the body. All this being said, let's look at some stats, get some facts, and get moving to a fit 'n' faith lifestyle.

We would first like to start out with a disclaimer. If you're a person of faith, we want to lead you to a passage that has been a default, a safety net if you will, for those who do not want to value physical exercise. 1 Timothy 4:8 says, "For physical training is of some value, but godliness has value for all things, holding promise for both the present life and the life to come." (NIV) *Some,* not <u>none</u>! It is *very* valuable to give glory to God by taking care of the most valuable possession He's given you on this earth – your body.

Exercise Defined – Activity requiring physical effort, carried out especially to sustain or improve health and fitness. (Oxford dictionary)

The reason we include this definition is that exercise doesn't mean being in a gym for hours or running a marathon. Exercise is multi-faceted. So, what are the various forms of exercise?

- Aerobic Movement – Sustained exercises that stimulate the heart and lungs (cycling, running, Zumba, various forms of dance, etc.).

- Anaerobic Movement – Short duration/high intensity exercise to promote muscle mass and strength. This could last from mere seconds to around two minutes (weightlifting, body weight movements such as push-ups, pull-ups, squats, etc.).

- Stretching – This would include:
  o Static stretching: extending a targeted muscle group to its maximum point and holding it for 15-30 seconds or more.
  o Dynamic stretching: for flexibility, you would use a continuous movement that mimics the exercise or sport that is to be performed.
  o Ballistic stretching: uses more of a bouncing movement to stretch a targeted muscle group. These stretches should always be done after static stretching to avoid injury.

- Balance and Agility – This includes dancing, skating, Zumba, and movements that mimic sports.

- High Intensity/Surge Training – Brief intervals of very intense work followed by a brief period of rest, repeated a certain number of times. Example: High intensity running in place for 10-20 seconds followed by a 10 second rest, repeated 3 to 10 times based on experience and fitness level.
  Or... do the following in 4 sets 3 times a day. This would make a HUGE impact on you physically:

    Do 4 sets of each of these, rapidly, with 10 repetitions.
    It will only take you 3-4 minutes:

      o 10 Squats
      o 10 Lifting alternate arms directly in front of you with palms down
      o 10 Jumping Jacks without jumping (just use the arm movements with legs out as if you did the jump)
      o 10 Shoulder presses above your head as if you are lifting weights

- Aquatics – Exercising in water lessens weight and pressure on the joints.

- Pilates – Focuses on the body's core (abdomen, obliques, back, inner and outer thighs, and buttocks/glutes).

There are many others. These are just a few examples. We list some websites you can check out for more details on the Resources page.

Some key benefits of exercise
1. Whole body detox (sweat!) + lymph system circulation (stretches & inversions!)
2. Reduces inflammation which is a leading cause of many diseases
3. Lowers type 2 diabetes risk
4. Slows down and/or reverses chronic illness
5. Lowers blood pressure
6. Improves mood (best anti-depressant and anxiety cure around!)
7. Increases bone density
8. Helps maintain brain function
9. Reduces the effects of stress and anxiety
10. Greatly reduces risk of stroke and heart attack

We like to say exercise makes you a palm tree instead of an oak tree. Let's face it; life is a series of calm and storm. When the storms come, the oak, as strong as it is, is hard and brittle. Its branches can snap easily in high winds. A palm tree, on the other hand, sways and, many times, stands strong even in hurricane force winds. Exercise makes you the palm tree that can withstand the winds of life by being flexible.

You say, "this is all good, but I don't have the time." Really? Take a minute right now to think of five of the most high-powered, active, fit, or influential people you can think of. Do you have them in mind?

Ok, now what do you have in common with them? We call it the 168 factor. You and every one of them *all* have 168 hours in a week – no more, no less. How you use (or mis-use) those hours reveals a priority problem, not a time scarcity problem. Make a chart with the number 168 at the top, and then subtract all the activities and "to do's" your life requires. I can almost guarantee you will have enough time leftover to exercise.

I (Mike) get up and do my workouts very early in the morning – 5:30 or 6am most days, but there are times when I don't feel disciplined enough to get on it right away. I have a tip that might help. This will bring conviction (hopefully) and some motivational guilt, if you will. Place your gym clothes, shoes, and goals list on top of your alarm clock or your phone if you use that as your alarm. This does it for me on those days when I'm tempted to opt out.

THE DANGERS OF NOT EXERCISING

The age of virtual living and remote everything is promoting a rapid excelling of every form of disease, especially in the chronic form. There is a half-truth being spread far and wide right now that says, "because of new drugs and technology, we're living longer." The other side of that is, because of not exercising we're also "dying longer." We don't hear much of that in the media or from Big Pharma companies. Many spend the last 5-15 years of their lives in a painful, disabling, chronic health crisis, or worse yet in bed in a nursing home. Is this what you want for your life? We think not. If this list puts fear into you, that's a good thing. If it puts fear into you enough to take immediate action, that's a greater thing, and it is the intention of what is stated below. The list is almost endless, but here are our top 5 dangers of not exercising:

1. Circulatory system problems – Your heart is a muscle just like any other in your body. Without use, it atrophies and weakens causing damage and a myriad of issues of which some are irreversible. In the United States and worldwide, cardiovascular disease is the number one killer (www.heart.org). The AHA (American Heart Association) reported in 2013, one in every three deaths in the United States was from heart disease, stroke, and other cardiovascular diseases.

2. Chronic diseases – Physical inactivity is a primary cause of many chronic diseases of which the list is just too long to include here, but here are a few: type-2 diabetes, hypertension, depression, anxiety, diverticulitis, asthma, arthritis.

105

3. Obesity (which leads to a variety of illnesses) – a whopping one third of the entire population in the world is overweight or obese. We normally think of the tragedy of health issues of the underweight in the world, but the sad truth is that early death comes more to the overweight than the underweight. Affluence and plenty can be two daggers in the quality and quantity of our lives.

4. Lack of energy and stamina, especially as you age.

5. Lack of mental focus and clarity – exercise oxygenates the body, especially the brain.

KEYS TO SUCCESS

There are many keys to success when it comes to getting started and being consistent with exercise. We will list a few of our favorites below:

1. Be a Kid Again – Author, pastor, and leadership teacher John Maxwell says that kids 0-7 are always asking "Why?", teenagers are always asking "Why not?", and grown-ups end up saying, "Just because." Be curious – take risks – don't give up!

2. Community – You are the sum of the people you choose to hang around most. Have an inner circle that has active lives that center around spiritual and physical wellness.

3. Find Your Target – Have time-framed, well-defined goals. As Zig Ziglar used to say, "If you aim at nothing, you'll hit it every time."

4. Mindset – You need positivity in your thinking and speaking. I (Mike) think P90x home workout creator and author Tony Horton says it best: "Stop saying I can't, and replace it by saying, 'I currently struggle with….'" You can do much more than you think. Line your thoughts and self-talk up with the potential of your capacity to achieve more.

5. Variety – As we said earlier in this chapter, exercise is more than just one thing. Find something you love to do, and then do it. What physical activity brought you joy as a youth? Weightlifting? Swimming? Another sport? Whatever it is, find it, dig it up, and go for it.

6. Get a Coach – Wherever you live, there are fitness coaches to be found. Many gyms offer short- or long-term fitness coaching. We offer online or one-on-one health & fitness coaching. Join a group or class that is both fun and challenging.

There is one "must have" piece of equipment that you already own that is vital for your success in fitness: a mirror! You, and only you decide each day whether or not you value the body God gave you, and what you will do with it. Exercise master, Jack LaLanne, was once asked by someone with deep curiosity, "Jack, what is the secret to your health and longevity?" His answer was a gem, for sure. "I've never woke up, sat on the end of the bed and felt a tap on my shoulder and a voice saying, 'Jack, sit back down and relax, I'll do this for you.'" His answer, simplified, was this: *action.* We never promote idolization of the body, but good stewardship, which is a Biblical principle, is going to take some action.

10

THE LEAN HORSE WINS THE RACE!

Sometimes one sentence can change the course of your journey. This was the case for me as I called in to a nutritional radio broadcast called Healthline. I (Mike) posed a question to host Dr. Bob Marshall (a man I highly respected) about several areas of wellness that I was struggling with. I gave him detail after detail about areas of change that I felt I needed. He agreed, but as he could see through the busyness of the details I gave him, he gave me a very simple, but profound answer. He simply said "Mike, the lean horse wins the race." In other words, you are over-thinking and over-burdening yourself with too many questions and details, and you're trying to do too much at once.

After the call, I took a long, hard look at my spiritual, emotional, mental, and physical life, and came to the conclusion that he was spot on. Isn't this true for so many of us? We are burdened down with too many thoughts, to do's, and comparisons, and we're trying to carry the weight of the world on our shoulders. This is also true with physical weight as well. Too much and we can't move smoothly through life. The input, whether it is about food, thoughts, or our schedule is just too much. It might be time to ask ourselves: "How much does my week weigh?" "Am I taking on so much that I can't focus in the areas that matter most?" "Just how much _____ am I putting in my body that is taking me down the road to disease?" Remember, the thief Jesus spoke of in John 10:10 wants it all. He doesn't care if you're caught up in comparison or bound and gagged by over-thinking and a busy schedule. Don't make agreements with him, and don't follow his systematic breakdown of your life and body. Identify the "criminals" that you are allowing into your life that steal your faith and fitness.

Stop making your life heavy. Dare to come alive and leave the trivial behind. As John Eldredge once put it, "it's suicide of the soul" not to awaken our hearts to their true desires. To awaken something means it must be aroused from its slumber. The priorities of your life may be slumbering because they're tired from being overcome by the urgency of the trivial. As Lillian often says to me personally, "It's time to wring out the sponge!" Well, maybe it's time for you to do the same?

PRIORITIES

John Maxwell unpacks the law of priorities in the "Leadership Bible" I am currently reading. He states that the Apostle "Paul narrowed his wedge and his focus to the *essentials.*" (*emphasis added*)

His secret? John refers to Philippians 3:7-14 (NIV):

[7] But whatever were gains to me I now consider loss for the sake of Christ. [8] What is more, I consider everything a loss because of the surpassing worth of knowing Christ Jesus my Lord, for whose sake I have lost all things. I consider them garbage, that I may gain Christ [9] and be found in him, not having a righteousness of my own that comes from the law, but that which is through faith in Christ—the righteousness that comes from God on the basis of faith. [10] I want to know Christ—yes, to know the power of his resurrection and participation in his sufferings, becoming like him in his death, [11] and so, somehow, attaining to the resurrection from the dead.

[12] Not that I have already obtained all this, or have already arrived at my goal, but I press on to take hold of that for which Christ Jesus took

hold of me. [13] Brothers and sisters, I do not consider myself yet to have taken hold of it. But one thing I do: Forgetting what is behind and straining toward what is ahead, [14] I press on toward the goal to win the prize for which God has called me heavenward in Christ Jesus.

1. He discerned what hindered him, meaning he let go of all the things *he* cherished, considering them distractions to grace.
2. He discovered what he wanted. Paul wanted God's righteousness, not his own. Christ became his solitary pursuit.
3. He determined how to get it. With single-minded passion, Paul forgot the past and pursued the prize of his call.

John then asks, as we do: Have you narrowed your focus? Can you list your priorities on one hand? What are you pursuing?

Without determination, you will be lured away from your path.

Your Assignment

Create a pie chart showing percentages per area of your life to see what pieces have gotten too much "pie."

Areas:
- spiritual
- physical
- relational
- emotional
- mental
- vocational
- recreational/hobbies
- self-improvement/self-care

Here's an example on the next page:

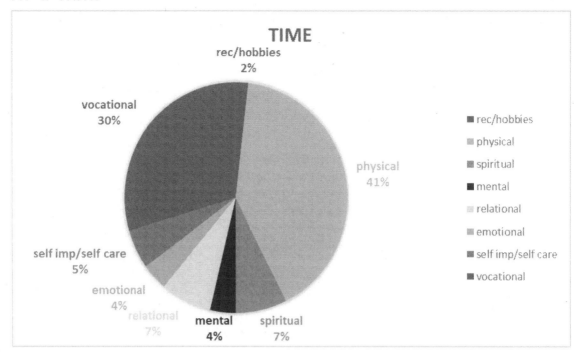

SUPERFOODS

If you want to be a lean horse that finishes the race, there are options available that you may not be aware of that can enhance your physical progress providing foods that can make a healthier you. Here are a few we would like to share:

It's commonly known that kale is a superfood. How about the following greens?

Superfoods That Are Even Healthier Greens Than Kale:

- **Romaine Lettuce**

    Romaine lettuce is a superfood that is healthier than kale. It is packed with high levels of folic acids, vitamin B, and vitamin K, which help to prevent high cholesterol levels. You can also find high levels of folate in romaine lettuce, which helps to fight off depression.

- **Parsley**

    Parsley is a great superfood that can help you meet your daily requirement of vitamin K. Parsley is also rich in vitamin C and offers

112

prevention from rheumatoid arthritis. Fresh parsley is recommended over dried because it possesses stronger flavor.

- **Collard Greens**

    Collard greens are well known for their ability to support the digestive system and make it healthy. Collard greens contain vitamins A, K, and C. These vitamins are essential to the body. Eating collard greens also helps you to lower high cholesterol, especially when they are steamed. For better results, select collard greens that are fresh. You can eat them raw or steam them lightly for about 5 minutes.

- **Spinach**

    Spinach provides a high amount of iron to your body. Iron is vital in maintaining muscle health and transporting oxygen throughout your body. Spinach contains a compound known as thylakoids that is found in the leaf membranes. This compound is an effective appetite suppressant, which helps to reduce food cravings and promotes healthy weight loss.

- **Watercress**

    Rich in vitamin B6, vitamin C, and beta carotene, watercress is a healthy superfood. It has the ability to prevent various cardiovascular illnesses. Its nutritional value and density are much greater than that of kale.

- **Chard**

    Chard offers protection against diabetes as it contains several polyphenol antioxidants that include anthocyanin, which also works as an anti-inflammatory. It works by regulating the glucose levels in your blood.

- **Leaf Lettuce**

    Leaf lettuce is another superfood that can be an alternative to kale. Two cups of leaf lettuce provide vitamin K that aids in keeping your bones strong and healthy. (Fitlife/superfoods)

If you thought that kale was the only "green" source of rich nutrients, now you have an added list of superfoods that are also incredible sources of nutrients and are even healthier than kale.

VITAMIN B17

B17, also known as laetrile and amygdalin, has been known to prevent or treat such health issues as kidney disease and various types of cancer. (Mercola/B17)

Vitamin B17 Foods

What are some vitamin B17 foods? There are quite a few, but many might not be what people would normally eat, particularly seeds. Fruit seeds have the highest concentration of B17 of any food, yet most people avoid eating them. There is some controversy surrounding vitamin B17 because it has cyanide molecules in it. In high doses cyanide is lethal, but the amounts found in food are required for proper health. Vitamin B17 in foods is the best and only way to get the vitamin into your body.

The best sources of B17 come from a variety of seeds, fruits, vegetables, sprouts, and nuts, and the very best source is found in apricot seeds. Soil and climate play a large role in how much vitamin B17 is in a particular food, so it can be difficult to determine the exact levels in each food. Below are some foods that are good sources of vitamin B17.

o **Fruit**

Many types of berries are a good source of this vitamin. Look for strawberries, huckleberries, cranberries, and blueberries. One serving (one cup) of gooseberries, blackberries, boysenberries, raspberries, and elderberries has 500 milligrams of vitamin B17. Other fruits that are good sources of the vitamin are peaches, plums, nectarines, cherries, and prunes, but remember, the pits in these fruits are the true sources of amygdalin.

o **Nuts**

Bitter almonds have the most B17, with cashews and macadamia nuts following.

o   **Leaves/Leafy Greens, Grasses**

Many leaves and grasses are a good source, but few people add them to their diet or have even heard of them. Johnson grass, Tunis grass, and arrow grass are good grasses to eat if you can find them. Alfalfa and eucalyptus leaves are better sources of B17; spinach, beet greens, and watercress all have moderate amounts.

o   **Sprouts**

Bamboo sprouts are the best sprouts to eat, but alfalfa, mung, and garbanzo sprouts are also decent sources.

o   **Seeds**

Apricot seeds are the best vitamin B17 source of any food. Other good seed sources include apples, grapes, berries, buckwheat, cherry, squash, and millet. Seeds can be added to salads and yogurt.

o   **Tubers**

Sweet potatoes and yams are much easier to come by at the grocery store, so when in doubt grab one of these. Plus, they're affordable!

Vitamin B17 – Foods Chart

Food Type	Examples
Fruit	Strawberries, huckleberries, cranberries, blueberries, gooseberries, blackberries, boysenberries, raspberries, elderberries, peaches, plums, nectarines, cherries, prunes
Nuts	Bitter almonds, cashews, macadamia nuts
Leaves/Leafy Greens/Grasses	Johnson grass, Tunis grass, arrow grass, alfalfa, eucalyptus, spinach, beet greens, watercress
Sprouts	Bamboo, alfalfa, mung, garbanzo
Seeds	Apricot, apples, grapes, berries, buckwheat, cherry, squash, millet
Tubers	Cassava, sweet potatoes, yams

How Much Vitamin B17 Is Appropriate to Consume?

People with cancer may want to use vitamin B17, even though the FDA does not regulate it. The basic consensus is that if you have a lot of cancer, you need a lot of B17, but be cautious and know that the side effects of large amounts of B17 are not properly documented. So before jumping from zero B17 to taking a mega-dose, perhaps consider incremental dosing to gauge how your body responds, and then you can add or subtract as determined by how you feel. It varies from person to person, but often 500 milligrams per day twice a day can be enough. Or try including some natural vitamin B17 foods listed on the previous page. (Doctorshealth/B17)

MORE SUPERFOODS

- **Sprouts**

  Sprouts, which are edible germinated seeds of flowers, beans, legumes, vegetables, or grains, are becoming well-known for their nutritional content and health benefits that you cannot get from their mature versions.

- **Brussels sprouts**

  Brussels sprouts are low in calories, and contain various vitamins (A, B1, B2, B6, C, and K), minerals (magnesium, phosphorus, iron, potassium, and calcium, to name a few), and antioxidants (ferulic and caffeic acids, kaempferol, and isorhamnetin). Brussels sprouts also contain sulfur-containing compounds called glucosinolates that break down into isothiocyanates and activate cancer-fighting enzymes.

  Brussels sprouts have always tested the patience of parents and the bravery of picky eaters, young and old. However, various types of sprouts are becoming well-known nowadays as a potent "superfood" that can do wonders for your body because they're rich in nutrients and deliver vital health benefits.

Cooked Brussels sprouts will have a bright green color, slightly crisp texture and nutty/sweet flavor. Don't overcook your Brussels sprouts as the taste changes and the nutrients become damaged. They will become overly smelly, mushy, and turn a pale green color.

- **Garlic**

     Garlic not only provides your food additional flavor and spice, but it's good for your health too. Its antioxidant properties can help suppress bacterial, viral and parasitic infections, fight free radicals and cancer cells, and improve your immune system. Garlic also helps reduce inflammation in your body and boost cardiovascular health and circulation.

- **Balsamic vinegar**

     While balsamic vinegar traces its roots to Italy, this ingredient has become popular in different cuisines worldwide because of its sweet and tart taste, which sets it apart from other types of vinegar. An article in *The Times of India* highlights balsamic vinegar's health benefits, including:

     o **Weight loss:** Balsamic vinegar helps in regulating your appetite, preventing overeating, and increasing the amount of time it takes for your stomach to empty. This vinegar is also low in calories and contains calcium, iron, manganese, and potassium.

     o **Helps blood circulation:** Antioxidants called polyphenols are present in balsamic vinegar, and they fix free radical-caused damage in your body. These polyphenols are also able to shield the body from heart disease and cancer.

     o **Helps in digestion:** Balsamic vinegar boosts the activity of an enzyme called pepsin. This enzyme enhances your body's metabolism and breaks down protein into smaller amino acids that could be absorbed more easily by your body.

     o **Improves immunity:** Balsamic vinegar is made from grapes, which contain antioxidants that are able to fight cell damage and enhance your body's immune system and flexibility of your blood platelets.

o **Regulates blood sugar:** If you're diabetic, balsamic vinegar is able to improve insulin sensitivity, and in turn normalizes blood sugar more easily and lessens unwanted diabetes side effects. (Mercola/balsamic)

SUPERFOODS: 5 BEST BITES FOR YOUR BUCK

1. **Blueberries (78 cents per serving)**
   THE CANCER-FIGHTING IMMUNITY BOOSTER
   - Contain cancer-fighting antioxidants for immunity
   - Increase metabolism and regulate blood sugar levels
   - Promote cell regeneration for healthy, youthful skin
   - Protect heart health and prevent osteoporosis
   - Support digestive health, weight loss, and circulation

2. **Cabbage (11 cents per serving)**
   THE BRAIN BEAST
   - Assists mental function and concentration
   - Helps dry up oily and acne skin
   - Supports stomach/digestive tract
   - Boosts immune system

3. **Sesame seeds (14 cents per serving)**
   THE IDENTITY PROTECTOR
   - Protect against cell/DNA damage
   - Promote reproductive health
   - Support blood health and muscle tone
   - Improve circulation and digestion

4. **Avocados (50 cents per serving)**
   THE LOVERS LINK

- Increase libido
- Boost heart health and reduce cholesterol/triglyceride levels
- Promote weight loss and satiety
- Increase absorption of fat-soluble nutrients (vitamin A, K, D, and E)

5. **Sweet potatoes (30 cents per serving)**
   THE GRAVITY DEFIER

- Help prevent sugar cravings
- Boost collagen production to combat premature aging
- Support stronger hair, skin, and nails
- Promote eye, bone, and immune system health
- Aid digestion and elimination (Wolfe/superfoods)

AVOCADO SEEDS

DON'T TRASH AVOCADO SEEDS: They're An Antioxidant-Filled Superfood

After cutting open a perfectly ripe avocado and scooping out the delicious flesh, what do you typically do with the seed?

Most people do not know that avocado seeds are edible as well. According to a study published in *Food Chemistry*, the seeds showed a "much higher antioxidant activity and phenolic content than the edible portions."

Here are **5 benefits of eating avocado seeds** that'll make you think twice the next time you move to throw them away:

1. **CONQUER CANCER CELLS** – Did you know that 70% of the antioxidants in avocados are found in the seeds? The seeds contain flavonol, a powerful antioxidant that helps to prevent and reduce tumor growth. A 2013 study published in *Pharmaceutical Biology*

found avocado extract from the flesh caused leukemia cells to self-destruct.

Move over berries, there's a new superfruit in town!

2. **DIMINISH DIGESTIVE ISSUES** – For centuries, avocado seeds have been used in South America to treat GI tract issues, including gastric ulcers, constipation, and diarrhea. These anti-inflammatory seeds contain more soluble fibers than most other foods on our planet! This superfruit is also sure to keep you full and help control blood sugar levels, so you are not reaching for a Kit Kat amidst a 3pm slump!

3. **HEAL YOUR HEART** – Avocados are an excellent source of heart-healthy monounsaturated fat, and thanks to their amino acid and dietary fiber content, the seeds can help lower cholesterol and prevent cardiovascular issues such as the formation of plaque, which can lead to strokes and heart attack.

   Dr. Tom Wu, who has earned the "World Famous Doctor" award from the United Nations for his breakthroughs with diabetes and cancer, says he *always* eats the seed and recommends heart disease patients do the same. "This soluble fiber binds to the fat and excess cholesterol. Then we can lower cholesterol and improve heart function naturally. Soluble fiber is tough to get in our diet. Oatmeal has some, but it cannot compare with the avocado seed."

4. **IMPROVE THE IMMUNE STRENGTH** – In flu season, it is important to know that avocado seeds are the perfect immune boosters, helping keep free radicals at bay and preventing bacterial, viral, and fungal infections!

5. **ALLEVIATE AGING** – The potent antioxidants in avocado seeds have been shown to slow down the aging process by rebuilding collagen, repairing cell damage, and improving the look and feel of your skin. In fact, you can even add avocado seed extract to your facial scrubs as a natural exfoliate! (Wolfe/avocado)

Surprised? I know we were when we were first introduced to superfoods and the value they are to the body.

FINAL THOUGHTS

The Unmoved Rock
– Author Unknown

Once upon a time, there was a man who was sleeping at night in his cabin when suddenly his room filled with light and the Savior appeared. The Lord told the man He had work for him to do, and showed him a large rock in front of his cabin. The Lord explained that the man was to push against the rock with all his might. This the man did, day after day. For many years he toiled from sun up to sun down, his shoulders set squarely against the cold, massive surface of the unmoving rock, pushing with all his might.

Each night the man returned to his cabin sore and worn out, feeling that his whole day had been spent in vain. Seeing that the man was showing signs of discouragement, Satan decided to enter the picture placing thoughts into the man's mind such as: "You have been pushing against that rock for a long time, and it hasn't budged. Why kill yourself over this? You are never going to move it." Thus giving the man the impression that the task was impossible and that he was a failure.

These thoughts discouraged and disheartened the man even more. "Why kill myself over this?" he thought. "I'll just put in my time, giving just the minimum of effort and that will be good enough." And that he planned to do until one day he decided to make it a matter of prayer and take his troubled thoughts to the Lord.

"Lord," he said, "I have labored long and hard in Your service, putting all my strength to do that which You have asked. Yet, after all this time, I have not even budged that rock a half a millimeter. What is wrong? Why am I failing?" To this the Lord responded compassionately, "My child, when long ago I asked you to serve Me and you accepted, I told you that your task was to push against the rock with all your strength, which you have done. Never once did I mention to you that I expected you to move it. Your task was to push.

"And now you come to Me, your strength spent, thinking that you have failed. But, is that really so? Look at yourself. Your arms are strong and muscled, your back sinewed and brown, your hands are callused from constant pressure, and your legs have become massive and hard. Through opposition, you have grown much and your abilities now surpass that which you used to have. Yet you haven't moved the rock. But your calling was to be obedient and to push and to exercise your faith and trust in MY wisdom. This you have done. I, My child, will now move the rock."

Keep pushing "your rock" my friends – We can do better!!! We do our part, and God will do the rest!

Live your life on purpose, centered on God, strengthened by His spirit, and quieted by His love. Be a lean horse and win the race!

As we wrap up this chapter, our prayer is that as you are finishing this book, it has, at the very least, caused you to be encouraged and rethink what is possible, and at the most, it has lit a fire for life change in you that will never be put out. There is so much more we could have included in this book, and there is so much more for you (and us) to continue learning. We hope you will connect with us on social media and/or the various avenues we provide for you to gain support and ongoing connection. We would love to hear from you.

11

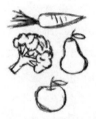

30-Day JUMPSTART
TO HEALTHY LIVING

30 Days to a New YOU!!

IT'S TIME FOR CHANGE!!! Overcome physical, emotional, and mental challenges, and jumpstart your healthy living journey!!!

<u>WHAT DO YOU NEED TO KNOW?</u>

Certain food groups (like sugar, grains, dairy, and legumes) could be having a negative impact on your health and fitness without you even realizing it. Are your energy levels inconsistent or non-existent? Do you have aches and pains that can't be explained by over-use or injury? Are you having a hard time losing weight no matter how hard you try? Do you have some sort of condition (like skin issues, digestive ailments, seasonal allergies, or fertility issues) that medication hasn't helped? These symptoms may be directly related to the foods you eat – even the "healthy" stuff. So how do you know if (and how) these foods are affecting you?

Strip them from your diet completely. Cut out all the psychologically unhealthy, hormone-unbalancing, gut-disrupting, inflammatory food groups for a full 30 days. Let your body heal and recover from whatever effects those foods may be causing. Push the "reset" button with your metabolism, systemic inflammation, and the downstream effects of the food choices you've been making. Learn once and for all how the foods you've been eating are actually affecting your day to day life and your long-term health.

The most important reason to keep reading?

This will change your life.

We cannot possibly put enough emphasis on this simple fact—the next 30 days will change your life. It will change the way you think about food, it will change your tastes, it will change your habits and your cravings. It could, quite possibly, change the emotional relationship you have with food and with your body. It has the potential to change the way you eat for the rest of your life. We know this because we did it, and many people have done so as well, and it changed our lives (and their lives) in a very permanent fashion. (Need convincing? Just read some of our stunning testimonials in Chapter 7 of this book.)

RULES

Eat Real Food

Eat tons of vegetables, some fruit, and plenty of good fats from fruits, oils, nuts, and seeds. Eat foods with very few ingredients, all pronounceable ingredients, or better yet, no ingredients listed at all because they're totally natural, organic, and unprocessed.

Avoid for 30 Days...

More importantly, here's what NOT to eat for the duration of your program. Omitting all of these foods and beverages will help you regain your healthy metabolism, reduce systemic inflammation, change your taste buds/palate, and help you discover how these foods are truly impacting your health, fitness, and quality of life.

- **Do not consume added sugar of any kind – real or artificial.** No maple syrup, honey, agave nectar, coconut sugar, Splenda, Equal, NutraSweet, xylitol, stevia, etc. Read your labels, because companies sneak sugar into products in ways you might not recognize.

- **Do not consume alcohol in any form, not even for cooking.** (And it should go without saying, but no tobacco products of any sort, either.)

- **Do not eat grains more than 2 times per week.** This includes (but is not limited to) wheat, rye, barley, oats, corn, rice, millet, bulgur, sorghum, amaranth, buckwheat, sprouted grains, or quinoa. This also includes all the ways we add wheat, corn, and rice into our foods in the form of bran, germ, starch, and so on. Again, read your labels.

- **Do not eat legumes more than 2 times per week.** This includes beans of all kinds (black, red, pinto, navy, white, kidney, lima, fava, etc.), chickpeas, lentils, and peanuts. No peanut butter, either. This also includes all forms of soy – soy sauce, miso, tofu, tempeh, edamame, and all the ways we sneak soy into foods (like lecithin).

- **Do not eat dairy.** This includes cow, goat, or sheep's milk products such as cream, cheese (hard or soft), kefir, yogurt (even Greek), and sour cream – with the exception of clarified butter or ghee. (See next page for details.)

- **Do not consume carrageenan, MSG, or sulfites.** If these ingredients appear in any form on the label of your processed food or beverage, it's out for the 30 days.

- **Do not try to re-create baked goods, junk foods, or treats with "approved" ingredients.** Continuing to eat your old, unhealthy food alternatives will affect your results. Remember, these are the same foods that got you into health-trouble in the first place and we want to change your palate.

One last and final rule: **You are not allowed to step on the scale or take any body measurements for the duration of the program (only once before you start and once when you end).** This is about so much more than weight loss, and to focus on your body composition means you'll miss out on the most dramatic and lifelong benefits this plan has to offer. So, no weighing yourself, analyzing body fat, or taking comparative measurements during your 30 days.

What else?

These foods are allowed during your 30-Day Program:

- **Clarified Butter or Ghee is best.** Clarified butter or ghee is the only source of dairy allowed during your 30 days. Plain old butter is NOT allowed, as the milk proteins found in non-clarified butter could impact the results of your program.
- **Fruit juice as a sweetener.** Some products or recipes will include fruit as a sweetener, which is fine for the purposes of the program – just don't overdo it. Dates and figs are great to have for that sweet taste you may long for but eat them rarely since they are high in natural sugar and calories.
- **Fruit.** It is not necessary during the 30 days, but, if you would like to see great weight loss, limit your fruit intake to 2 servings per day and choose fruit that is lower on the glycemic index.
- **Certain legumes.** Green beans are fine, as well as sugar snap peas and snow peas. While they're technically a legume, these are far more "pod" than "bean," and green plant matter is generally good for you. Other legumes are okay <u>2 times a week</u>.
- **Vinegar.** Most forms of vinegar, including white, balsamic, apple cider, red wine, and rice vinegar are allowed during your program. The only exceptions are vinegars with added sugar, or malt vinegar, which generally contains gluten. Check your labels.
- **Salt** (use sea salt only – a Himalayan pink sea salt is recommended). Did you know that all iodized table salt contains sugar? Sugar (often in the form of dextrose) is chemically essential to keep the potassium iodide from oxidizing and being lost. Because all restaurant and pre-packaged foods contain salt, we're making salt an exception to our "no added sugar" rule.

THIRTY DAYS

For 30 straight days. Your job? **Eat Good Food.**

The only way this will work is if you give it the full thirty days: no cheats, slips, or "special occasions." This is a fact, you need such a small amount of any of these inflammatory foods to break the healing cycle—one bite of pizza, one splash of milk in your coffee, one lick of the spoon mixing the batter within the 30 day period and you've broken the "reset" button, requiring you to start over again on Day 1.

You must commit to the full program, exactly as written. Anything less and we make no claims as to your results or the chances of your success. Anything less and you are selling yourself—and your potential results—short.

It's For Your Health

This is for those of you who are considering taking on this life-changing month but aren't sure you can actually pull it off, cheat free, for a full 30 days. This is for the people who have tried this before but who "slipped" or "fell off the wagon" or "just HAD to eat (fill in food here) because of this (fill in event here)." This is for you. You can do this! We have seen so many others do it and reap the benefits – YOU can too!!!

- **It is going to be hard, but getting a disease or being depressed is even harder – yes?** Beating cancer is hard. Birthing a baby is hard. Losing a parent is hard. Be encouraged! You've done harder things than this, so... remember to skip the excuses altogether. You can complete the program as written. It's only thirty days, and it's for the most important health cause on earth – the only physical body you will ever have in this lifetime.

- **Don't even consider the possibility of a "slip."** There is no "slip." You make a choice to eat something unhealthy. It is always a choice, so do not phrase it as if you had an accident/slip. Commit to the program 100% for the full 30 days. Don't give yourself an excuse to fail before you've even started.

- **You never, ever, ever have to eat anything you don't want to eat.** Learn to say no. Learn to change your thinking about food and give yourself the gift of a "no, thank you" for yourself. Just because it's your sister's birthday, or your best friend's wedding, or your company picnic does not mean you have to eat anything. It's always a choice, and we hope you are able to stop succumbing to peer pressure.

- **This does require effort.** Grocery shopping, meal planning, planning ahead for dining out, explaining the program to friends and family, and dealing with stress will all prove challenging at some point during your program. You have all the tools, guidelines, and resources you'll need, but take responsibility for your own plan. Improved health, fitness, and quality of life don't happen automatically – it will take one good choice after the other.

- **You can do this.** You've come too far to back out now. You want to do this. You need to do this. And we believe that you can do this. So stop thinking about it, and start doing. Right now, this very minute, tell someone that you are starting the program.

Finally...

We want you to participate. We want you to take this seriously and see amazing results in unexpected areas. Even if you don't believe this will actually change your life, if you're willing to give it 30 short days, it will...it truly will. It is that important – YOU are that important.

WHERE TO START

Clean House

First, get the stuff you won't be eating out of the house. Having tempting food sitting around is a recipe for failure – so let's put some distance between you and those snacks, shall we? Time to clean out the pantry – toss the stuff you won't be eating, give it to a neighbor, or donate it to a local food bank, as long as it's not within reach when the temptation hits. Habit research shows that the average craving lasts only 3-5 minutes, which means by the time you change out of your PJs, find your keys, grab your wallet, and head for the door, the craving has passed, and you've stuck to your plan another day.

Create Non-visible Spaces

If you're the only one at home doing the 30, chances are your family isn't going to take kindly to you tossing their favorite snacks and desserts. Dedicate one drawer in your fridge and an out-of-the-way cabinet for these off-plan items, so you don't have to reach around the Oreos every time you need a can of coconut milk.

Plan a Week's Worth of Meals

If you're a busy bee or just a super-planner, get ahead of the game by writing down a week's worth of breakfasts, lunches, and dinners.

Remember, meals can be so simple, no recipe is required—just take healthy ingredients and make them a meal. A smoothie is the perfect way to make an entire meal that is nourishing and filling.

Go Shopping

Time to stock up on healthy foods! Use your meal plan to help you create a shopping list (we have included a great list in the Appendix of healthy foods to purchase), and head to your local grocery store, health food store, farmers market, or co-op.

- Load up on vegetables and fruit (prioritizing vegetables). Although many produce items are now available year-round, shop seasonally for the best price and taste or purchase frozen organic.
- Next up—healthy fats, like extra-virgin olive oil, coconut oil, avocado, pastured butter (to clarify at home), olives, nuts, and seeds.
- Finally, stock your pantry with the essentials—and don't forget to check Amazon.com or other online stores such as SwansonVitamins.com or Vitacost.com for not-necessary-but-nice-to-have items you may not be able to find locally.

Take Action!

Unless you plan on living like a hermit for the next 30 days, your program will likely be littered with obstacles. Unfortunately, when we hit some of these, we often quit. Why? Because we have no *plan*.

So instead, think about the next 30 days and anticipate your obstacles. Then, make a plan for what you'll do when you face them.

Prepare, Prepare, Prepare Some More

First, write down every potential stressful, difficult, or complicated situation you may encounter during your 30 days. These may include business lunches, family dinners, travel plans, a long day at work, birthday parties, holiday celebrations, or office gatherings.

Next, create an if/then plan for each potentially difficult situation: "If this happens, then I'll do this." Here are some examples:

- **Business lunch:** If my co-workers give me a hard time about not ordering a drink, then I'll say, "I'm doing this food experiment right now to see if I can make my allergies better (you're allergic to bad food – ☺ – we all are), so it's mineral water with lime for me tonight."
- **Family dinner:** If my Mom expresses concern about this "crazy diet" I'm on, then I'll say, "I'm not dieting, Mom—I'm eating lots of healthy food, and I'm really not missing out on anything. In fact, let me bring dessert!"
- **Travel day**: If I get to the airport and my flight is delayed, then I'll snack on the apples, carrot sticks, and the small packet of almond butter I brought in my carry-on. Note: see https://www.tsa.gov/travel/security-screening/whatcanibring/food for details on what's allowed.
- **Long day at the office**: If I get home from work starving and cranky and I'm tempted to order take-out, then I'll pick a meal from my go-to list.*

  ➤ *Plan three quick and easy "go-to" meals you can make in ten minutes or less, with foods you always have on hand.*

Take Action!
- Create your plan
- Create your three "go-to" meals
- Stock up on emergency food for your car, gym bag, and/or office

You may need just a day or two to prepare, or you may need a week or two to get your house (and your head) around the changes you're about to introduce. There is no perfect timeline—you'll have to decide what works best for you.

Start Date

Here are some general guidelines:

- Start *as soon as you possibly can*, given the amount of preparation time you need.
- If you've got a once-in-a-lifetime vacation, an international trip to an unfamiliar location, or a wedding (especially your own!) in your imminent future, consider starting the 30 *after* those events. Navigating the 30 for the first time under those conditions may prove extremely difficult, and we don't want you to begin your program stressed out.
- If you've got a family dinner, a business lunch, or a bridal shower in your imminent future, consider it an opportunity to take your program skills out on the town! You'll have to deal with lots of new situations during your program, so write these events into your plan for the month, but *don't* let them push it off.

Go Public!

Once you've decided and made the commitment, tell someone! Anyone! Everyone! Write your start date on the whiteboard at work, create a 30-Day countdown calendar, or post on your Facebook page, Twitter, or Instagram feed.

Congratulations! You are now officially part of the 30-Day Program!

SUPPLEMENTS & SUCH FOR THE JOURNEY

- ■ Whole Body Detox kit (you will start on Day 1)
- ■ Digestive enzymes (taken with any cooked food)
- ■ Probiotics
- ■ Milled flaxseed

- Multi-vitamin included in a plant-based protein powder
     OR multi-vitamin in pill or liquid form (making sure it is from a whole food source and water soluble) PLUS a separate plant-based protein powder
- Omega 3's – Krill Oil or Flaxseed Oil in capsules or liquid
- Vitamin D3 (5,000 - 8,000 IUs)
- Vitamin B complex with C
- Curcumin
- Lithium Orotate & 5-htp (minerals that are only taken by those with depression and not on anti-depressants)

Get Moving!
5 – 10 minutes each day: stretch, surge, walk
3 times a week: 60-minute workout (or break it up into two 30-minute workouts in a day)

Food/Groceries (see list on next page for what to purchase ONLY organic)
- buy produce for 1 – 2 green smoothies per day
- kale, spinach, collard, romaine – dark greens
- celery, carrots, cucumbers, squash, peppers, etc.
- fruit – (check the glycemic index if one of your goals is weight loss)
- green apples – eat 1 a day; a banana a day is good too
- frozen organic fruit for smoothies
- cold pressed coconut oil
- apple cider vinegar (with mother)
- quinoa, brown or black rice
- walnuts, almonds, pine nuts, cashews (raw only – no dry roasted) – consume only ¼ cup a day of nuts and seeds for best results
- seeds – pumpkin, sunflower, chia, hemp
- beans – black, kidney, navy, pinto, lentil
- veggie broth
- steel cut oats
- water – reverse osmosis – filtered – clean, free from fluoride and chlorine

❖ toothpaste with NO fluoride or make your own from 2 parts coconut oil to 1 part baking soda (only the type without aluminum) and 20 drops of peppermint essential oil or thieves essential oil blend

Buy Organic Only

Apples	Snap peas
Peaches	Potatoes
Nectarines	Hot peppers
Strawberries/All Berries	Kale and Collard greens
Grapes	Cucumbers
Tomatoes	Sweet bell peppers
Celery	Spinach

There is so much you get to enjoy on this program – many things that you CAN have that will be nutritious and yummy. You will not be hungry, and your taste buds will change. So...what else can you have that we will help you with?

Veggies – any kind – there will be lots of creative ideas and recipes both in this book and on our Facebook page: *LifeCare – Living Well: Health & Wellness group*. In these recipes, you'll find a variety of spices, and the stir fry meals are great!! Yum!

Did we say you can have lots of veggies? Yes! You can have TONS of veggies!! Awesome, yummy soups (bean, veggie, split-pea), roasted veggies, raw veggies for snacks, and some fruit.

Smoothies – you can have smoothies as a meal or as a treat – wait till you try some of these!! YUM!

Emotional/Spiritual

Journal Your Journey – At the end of every day, write at least a sentence or two about what you are experiencing – physically, emotionally, mentally, and spiritually.

Accountability & Encouragement – Be sure to connect with the others you are on this 30-Day Journey with – create and use a Facebook group as often as you can to encourage, ask for prayer, etc., or join our Health Page.

READY, GET SET, GO!

Begin Your 30-Day Journey!

We are already praying for your 30-Day Journey and the transformation that is going to happen!!! WOW – just wait – body, soul, spirit transformation!!

SAMPLE FOOD PLAN FOR 30-DAY JUMPSTART

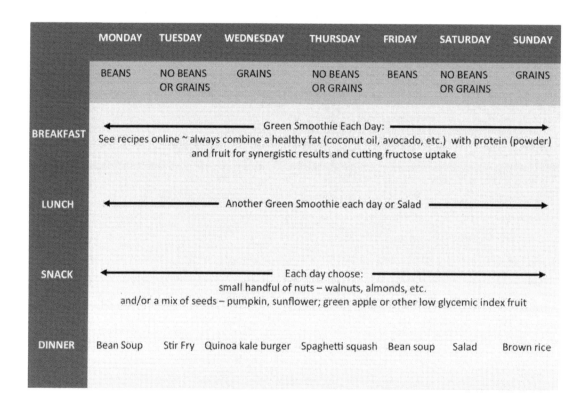

	MONDAY	TUESDAY	WEDNESDAY	THURSDAY	FRIDAY	SATURDAY	SUNDAY
	BEANS	NO BEANS OR GRAINS	GRAINS	NO BEANS OR GRAINS	BEANS	NO BEANS OR GRAINS	GRAINS
BREAKFAST	\<-- Green Smoothie Each Day: --> See recipes online ~ always combine a healthy fat (coconut oil, avocado, etc.) with protein (powder) and fruit for synergistic results and cutting fructose uptake						
LUNCH	\<-- Another Green Smoothie each day or Salad -->						
SNACK	\<-- Each day choose: --> small handful of nuts – walnuts, almonds, etc. and/or a mix of seeds – pumpkin, sunflower; green apple or other low glycemic index fruit						
DINNER	Bean Soup	Stir Fry	Quinoa kale burger	Spaghetti squash	Bean soup	Salad	Brown rice

Important information for those dealing with depression and looking for alternatives/ a way to boost/change mood.

What is the cause of depression?

Depression doesn't discriminate. It can affect anyone at any stage of life, even if life seems to be going well. Research has shown that brain chemistry, genetics, personalities, and environmental factors can all play a role in causing depression.

- **Brain chemistry:** Serotonin and norepinephrine are chemicals in the brain that affect our mood. If these chemicals are not being produced or affected by some sort of abnormality, they can cause symptoms of depression or anxiety. Many times, chemical imbalance is caused by the prevalent toxic chemicals in things we eat. Processed foods, not to mention BPA-laced cans and food packaging, are loaded with chemicals that affect our hormones. Refined sugar and sugar substitutes also play a major role in disrupting normal communication with the brain.
- **Genetics:** If someone in your family has depression, you might have a predisposition to it.
- **Personality:** Sometimes personalities can make a person more vulnerable to depression. For example, people who are more pessimistic, tend to be overwhelmed by stress, or have low self-esteem are at an increased risk for depression.
- **Environmental factors:** If a person resides in an environment that constantly exposes them to violence, abuse, neglect, or poverty, they can become more susceptible to depression.
- **Other causes:** Medical conditions such as a brain tumor or a vitamin deficiency can cause depression. There are also specific types of depression, such as post-partum depression experienced by new mothers.

How can you help manage depression in a healthy way?

The National Institute of Mental Health states, "Depression, even the most severe cases, can be effectively treated." That's great news. But is there an alternative to popping pills like Prozac or Paxil?

As described above, one of the top reasons why people become depressed is due to a chemical imbalance. As with all illnesses and health conditions, your body functions at its best when it's supported by a strong army of raw nutrients while simultaneously freeing itself of toxins.

Focusing on the right nutrition from a plant-based diet is the most effective way to live a healthier lifestyle and get your body the vitamins and minerals it needs to stave off depression. (Hallelujah/depression)

It's time to change what you put in your body using our basic health principles—starting by eating raw, plant-based foods, juices/raw food smoothies, and pure supplements—the most effective way to ensure that you get the right nutrition to effectively prevent and manage depression.

EMOTIONAL/MENTAL & SPIRITUAL HEALTH – WEEKLY EXERCISES

WEEK ONE

Read and meditate on the story of the rich young man in Matthew 19 and on Mark 8:34. With Jesus, if we want to gain anything worthwhile, we must give up. If we want to be filled, we must deny ourselves. If we want to truly get close to God, we'll have to distance ourselves from things that hinder that. If we want to conquer our cravings, we'll have to redirect them to God. Journal what God speaks to you as you read.

Do this for the next 7 days:

Consider a problem you face. On a scale from 1-10 (10 meaning you will do anything to solve your problem, and 1 meaning you will blame the situation on others for your problem), where would you put yourself today? Take a moment to think about this honestly. Where you place yourself on this scale is entirely up to you. You have no reason to exaggerate or to be overly hard on yourself.

What will you be doing differently when you move to the next number on the scale? Write your answers in your journal. For example, if you believe you are at a 5, what will you be doing differently today when you are at a 6? It is important to think of this in as concrete a fashion as possible. You want to create a vision of your future where you are taking greater action to solve your own problems with God's help. If you were being videotaped as you begin to act on your next number up the scale, what would we see you doing differently? You may be tempted to say what you would not be doing; "I would not be yelling or being so negative or reaching for the donut or reaching for the latte or I would not be so angry." Okay, so...what will you do instead? How exactly will you be doing this? Your primary concern will be how you will be doing something differently – not what anyone else is doing, and **not** what you **won't** be doing.

As your 7 days progress, what do you observe? Write everything down.

Congrats! It has been a week. On to week #2.

WEEK TWO

Do this for the next 7 days:

We all have challenges, difficulties, problems. Remember that whatever the problem may be that is concerning you, this problem does not happen all the time. There are good times. There are parts of your life that you are happy with. Take a moment to consider how these good or better things are happening. What are you doing differently in those areas? What are you doing and what will you continue to do to have these good things happen and to build on them? Write down, at the end of your day, what strengths you have that helped these "better" times to happen each day.

It is God's intention for you to succeed – but keep in mind that His definition of success may be different than yours, and His is the only one that really counts. You can bring yourself in agreement with HIS intention. One of the most important areas to succeed in as far as God is concerned is in the area of relationships. When your intention is for others, and you deliberately work toward being a blessing and helping others succeed, you are living out one of God's intentions for you. If a person you are relating with is not very likable, keep in mind that you have not always been very likable from God's point of view. Make a choice to stop focusing on other people as "problems." Instead, recognize the problem as the problem. Do the same for your issues/problems. Each day – rate yourself 1-10 on whether or not you are a strong part of God's team in bringing positive change to yourself and your world/others, and then respond to the following: How will you be adjusting your actions and reactions? What do you notice that is different with the interaction? What works better than what you were doing previously? – Do more of it! Write down what occurs when you are more in agreement with God's plan.

WEEK THREE

Here is your next assignment:

Get a small business card and write the word POWER on the back. Draw a line under the word power and write the word WISDOM. Keep this card in your pocket and remove it only when you begin to blame someone for something. Then take out the card and imagine yourself giving it away to that person you are blaming. Remind yourself through this action that you are beginning to give away your power and strength in Jesus Christ – and with it your wisdom to know what to do next.

Write down what you noticed about yourself and others when you did this. You can stop blaming by seeing this person and situation as a part of your personal growth. Then you will assume your responsibility to learn from God. As you do this, you will reclaim the card and put it back in your pocket. Again, write down what you noticed when you did this. How did your interaction with the person or persons change? Repeat what has been working well for you.

WEEK FOUR/FINAL WEEK

For this week/your final week: You were previously asked to Journal Your Journey for the 30 days. This week – if you are part of our Facebook group, post on that page at least one of your entries to encourage one another as you near the end of the 30 Days. Post in each of the four areas of what you have experienced. If you are not part of the Facebook group yet, we would love to have you join (see the Resources page in the Appendix).

Here is what you were supposed to be journaling: At the end of every day write at least a sentence or two about what you are experiencing:

1. physically
2. emotionally
3. mentally
4. spiritually

APPENDIX

RECIPES

(Note: all * recipes can be used during the 30-Day Program)

SMOOTHIES

Super Charged Key Lime Pie Smoothie

2 cups full-fat organic coconut milk

½ cup soaked cashews

2 Tbsp of raw honey

½ avocado

1 large handful of spinach

Juice of one lime

1 frozen banana

¼ tsp vanilla

Servings: 1 Smoothie

*Detox Drink (eliminate stevia for 30-Day Program)

Total Time: 2 minutes   Serves: 1

INGREDIENTS

1 glass of filtered water (12-16 oz.)

2 Tbsp apple cider vinegar

2 Tbsp lemon juice

1 tsp cinnamon

1 dash Cayenne Pepper (optional)

stevia to taste

Directions:

Blend all ingredients together

Smoothie options to try: eliminate the stevia or sweetener on any that call for that for the 30-Day Program, and even try to leave out things that you might not have on hand and just try them.

*Choc-Banana Smoothie Bowl

The combination of cacao, coconut and maca makes this the perfect mood-boosting and hormone-balancing bowl of goodness. Plus, it tastes just like a bowl of chocolate and banana ice cream, so why wouldn't you be happier after eating this?

INGREDIENTS

1 frozen banana

½ cup coconut milk

1 Tbsp cacao powder

1 Tbsp shredded coconut

1 Tbsp coconut oil

½ Tbsp maca powder

1 tsp vanilla

1 tsp cinnamon

1 tsp chia seeds

2 dates (pitted)

Blend everything together in your blender and enjoy this one in a bowl, just like you are enjoying a bowl of ice cream...only 10 times better!

*The Green Mood Booster

INGREDIENTS

1 frozen banana

1 handful of spinach

½ avocado

2 Tbsp nut butter

1 tsp vanilla

1 cup almond milk

½ cup coconut water

Greens (any kind – spinach, kale)

3 Tbsp raw cacao nibs

Blend everything (except raw cacao nibs). Once the smoothie is nice and smooth, add in cacao nibs and give another blend. We like to still have a little crunch in these, and it's nice to sprinkle some on top! Enjoy.

Don't let those cravings win you over with chocolate and sweets, use these cravings as an excuse to make a beautiful berry smoothie like this one. The addition of cacao powder will give you an extra boost of happiness while also feeding your chocolate craving.

*Berry-Rich Craving Saver
INGREDIENTS

½ cup blueberries

3 - 5 strawberries, depending on size and freshness

1 cup coconut milk

½ avocado

1 Tbsp goji berries

1 Tbsp cacao powder (optional)

2 tsp ground flaxseed

1 tsp chia seeds

Blend everything together until totally smooth and enjoy!

*Pumpkin Coconut Paleo Smoothie Recipe
Serves: 2

1 cup pumpkin purée (organic or make your own from scratch is best)

1 cup coconut milk (full fat, not light)

1 frozen banana

2 Tbsp almond butter

cinnamon

Instructions:

Place all ingredients in the blender and blend until smooth.

*Chocolate Banana Nut Smoothie Recipe

Total Time: 2 minutes   Serves: 1

INGREDIENTS

1 cup coconut milk

⅓ cup sprouted almond butter

1 banana, peeled

2 Tbsp cacao powder

2 cup ice cubes

stevia to taste

Directions:

Place all ingredients in a blender and blend until desired consistency is reached.
Serve immediately.

One of the easiest ways to give your day a swift nutritional kick first thing in the AM? Sipping down a smoothie. Whether you're breaking your cleanse or just keeping your body strong, there is a smoothie concoction perfect for every morning.

*Carrot Mango Coconut

1 large carrot (grated), 1 cup frozen mango, 1 - 2 Tbsp unsweetened shredded coconut. Blend with ½ to 1 cup liquid.

*Cherry Blueberry Kale

1 cup kale, 1 cup cherries, ½ cup blueberries. Blend with ½ to 1 cup liquid.

*Cherry Mango Yogurt

1 cup diced mango, 1 cup frozen cherries, ½ cup plain unsweetened yogurt. Blend with ½ to 1 cup liquid.

*Ginger Pina Colada

2 cups frozen pineapple, 1 lime (peeled and sliced), ½ inch piece of ginger (thinly sliced). Blend with ½ to 1 cup liquid.

*Raspberry Banana Chia

1 ½ cups frozen raspberries, 1 large banana (sliced), 1 Tbsp chia seeds. Blend with ½ to 1 cup liquid.

*Cranberry Pineapple Spinach

1 ½ cups pineapple, ½ cup cranberries, 1 cup spinach. Blend with ½ to 1 cup liquid. (Can substitute another berry for the cranberries.)

*Banana Blueberry Chocolate

1 large banana (sliced), 1 cup blueberries, 1 Tbsp cocoa or cacao powder. Blend with ½ to 1 cup liquid.

*Tangerine Pineapple Banana

2 tangerines (peeled and segmented), ½ cup frozen pineapple, 1 frozen banana. Blend with ½ to 1 cup liquid.

*Peanut Butter Strawberry

1 cup frozen strawberries, 1 large banana (sliced), 1 - 2 Tbsp peanut butter. Blend with ½ to 1 cup liquid.

*Mango Berry Coconut

1 cup mixed berries, 1 cup mango, 2 Tbsp unsweetened shredded coconut. Blend with ½ to 1 cup liquid.

*Green Swiss Chard Smoothie

by Jim Perko, YouBeauty Culinary Expert

Servings: 5

INGREDIENTS

2 cups cleaned swiss chard, stems removed, leaves roughly chopped, firmly packed

1 cup green seedless grapes

1 Bartlett pear, core, stem and seeds removed

1 orange, peeled and quartered

2 bananas, peeled

1 tsp chia seeds

¼ cup water

2 cups ice

*Kale, Pineapple and Coconut Milk Smoothie

By Heather Bauer, R.D.   Servings: 2

INGREDIENTS

1 scoop Vanilla Whey Protein Powder (use a plant-based powder for 30-Day)

½ cup unsweetened coconut milk or coconut water

2 cups baby kale or baby spinach

1 ½ cups chopped pineapple

1 ripe banana, frozen, broken into chunks

Ice

Berry Protein Bash

Servings: 2

This is one of our favorite combos – strawberries, blueberries, and banana. We up the protein by adding almonds. We also love the extra dietary fiber and vitamin E from the almonds.

INGREDIENTS

2 cups spinach, fresh

2 cups almond milk, unsweetened

1 cup strawberries

1 cup blueberries

1 banana

½ cup almonds*

Directions:

1. Blend spinach and almond milk until smooth.

2. Next add the remaining fruits and blend again.

Soak almonds overnight in water before blending, or use almond meal instead. Use at least one frozen fruit to make the green smoothie cold. Any variety of berry can be substituted.

*Immunity Green Smoothie

By Katrine van Wyk, author of "Best Green Drinks Ever"

Servings: 1

INGREDIENTS

1 cup coconut water

2 leaves romaine lettuce

½ green apple, such as Granny Smith

¼ cucumber

¼ avocado, peeled

½ lemon, peeled

½-inch slice fresh ginger

½ cup fresh parsley

1 serving probiotic powder or the contents of a probiotic capsule (follow instructions on the bottle)

3 - 4 ice cubes, optional

Frozen Green Lemonade

By Katrine van Wyk, author of "Best Green Drinks Ever"

Servings: 1

INGREDIENTS

½ cup chilled mint tea

½ cup spinach

½ cup or 2 leaves romaine lettuce

5 mint leaves

1 lemon, peeled

5 drops or 1 packet Stevia

1 cup ice

Nut Butter Chocolate

1 ½ cups almond milk (unsweetened)

Half a spoon of cacao powder

Half a spoon of almond butter

banana

cinnamon

Vanilla protein powder

Calories: around 400-420

*you could add coconut oil or flax seeds if you want

Smoothie

1 cup baby spinach

1 orange (peeled)

½ cup carrot

1 Tbsp milled flaxseed

1 scoop Protein Powder

3 frozen strawberries

½ cup almond milk (unsweetened)

¼ cup filtered water

Consistency via blender: medium

Makes 16 oz. (2 cups) blended

*Chocolate Cherry Green Smoothie

Author: Dreamy Leaf

INGREDIENTS

1 cup plant or nut milk

3 Tbsp raw cacao

1 cup (or more) pitted cherries - you can use frozen

½ avocado (can sub ½ frozen banana)

1 big handful of spinach

1 Tbsp chia seeds

3 Tbsp hemp seeds, optional for extra protein and healthy fats

dash of cinnamon

Instructions:

Throw all ingredients in a high power blender and blend until smooth.

*For a sweeter smoothie, add in a pitted Medjool date.

<u>Juice</u> – Great Juice to create with your juicer if you have one!

Ginger

Lemon

Kale

2 green apples

Carrots

Half a zucchini

Kiwi

Orange

* this is around 100 calories after it's been juiced, and it tastes great!

COFFEE CREAMER

Kerrygold brand butter (which is organic grass fed) and organic coffee grounds, cinnamon and a small amount of honey. 120 calories, mainly because of the butter which is 100 per tablespoon.

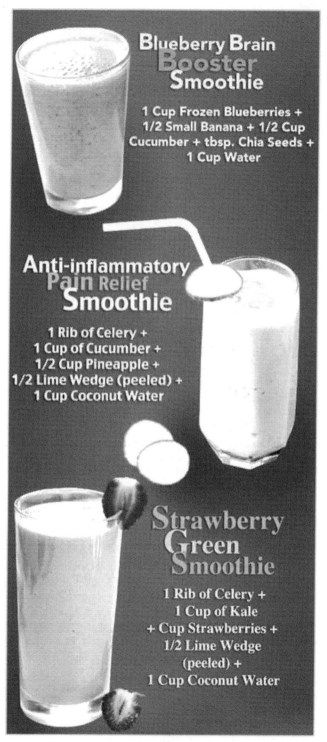

Blueberry Brain Booster Smoothie

1 Cup Frozen Blueberries +
1/2 Small Banana + 1/2 Cup
Cucumber + tbsp. Chia Seeds +
1 Cup Water

Anti-inflammatory Pain Relief Smoothie

1 Rib of Celery +
1 Cup of Cucumber +
1/2 Cup Pineapple +
1/2 Lime Wedge (peeled) +
1 Cup Coconut Water

Strawberry Green Smoothie

1 Rib of Celery +
1 Cup of Kale
+ Cup Strawberries +
1/2 Lime Wedge
(peeled) +
1 Cup Coconut Water

MAIN DISHES

*Stir Fry (Eliminate egg for 30-Day Program)

brown rice

broccoli

red pepper

yellow zucchini

mushrooms

kale

garlic

celery

1 egg

Prepare brown rice separately according to package directions. Combine all other ingredients in a frying pan with a healthy oil, then add the egg at the end as you continue to stir. Add cooked brown rice.

*Stir Fry

grapeseed oil

mushrooms

broccoli

garlic

green onions

yellow pepper

kale

pine nuts

ginger powder

sea salt and cayenne pepper to taste

*Interesting Soup

sweet dumpling squash

vegetable stock

a little bit of unsweetened coconut milk

ginger

sea salt

cinnamon

nutmeg

Creamy Vegan Corn Chowder

Prep time: 5 mins   Cook time: 25 mins   Total time: 30 mins

A quick, simple and healthy soup made with corn, potatoes, celery and red pepper.

Author: Crazy Vegan Kitchen   Serves: 4

INGREDIENTS

1 Tbsp olive oil

1 yellow onion, diced

1 red pepper, diced

2 sticks of celery, diced

1 medium potato, peeled and diced

3 Tbsp almond flour

1 cup almond/oat milk

2 cups vegetable broth

1 tsp celery salt

1 tsp smoked paprika

1 tsp dried parsley

4 ears of corn, shucked

1 tsp apple cider vinegar

salt/pepper, to taste

chopped green onion, for garnish

cilantro, for garnish

extra bits of corn and red pepper, for garnish

Instructions:

In a large pot, heat olive oil. Sauté onion, red pepper and celery for 10 min or until soft. Add diced potato and mix well. Once mixed, add in flour and stir to coat veggies. Cook for a minute or two before adding your non-dairy milk of choice and vegetable broth. Add celery salt, smoked paprika, and dried parsley into the pot. Stir well and then bring to a boil. Once at a boil, reduce to simmer, cover pan with a lid and simmer gently for 15 - 20 minutes, or until potato bits are tender.

Once potato is tender, add shucked corn kernels and stir to combine. Let cook for another 5 - 10 minutes or until corn is tender to your liking.

Transfer ¼ - ⅓ of the soup to a blender (depending on how thick you want the chowder) and blend till smooth. Pour back into the pot and stir well. (Or use an immersion blender.)

Stir in apple cider vinegar and taste to adjust seasoning before serving. Top with chopped green onion, cilantro and extra bits of corn/red pepper.

*Avocado Cashew Soup
Servings: 2
1 avocado
1 organic cucumber
2 green onions, chopped
juice of 1 lime
1 tsp of pink salt
1 cup of cashew cream

Instructions:
<u>To Make Cashew Cream</u>:   1 cup cashews   1 cup water
Soak 1 cup cashews in cold water for two hours.
Drain cashews and rinse.
Place in blender with 1 cup water.
Blend on high for several minutes until creamy.

<u>To Make Soup</u>:
1. For the soup, chop cucumber, avocado, and green onions and combine with 1 cup cashew cream in a blender or food processor.
2. Add lime juice, salt, and pepper and blend until smooth. Garnish with fresh tomatoes, cilantro, or avocado slices.

*Red Lentil Soup with Lemon

Servings: 4   Time: 45 minutes

This is a lentil soup that defies expectations of what lentil soup can be. It is light, spicy and a bold red color (no murky brown here): a revelatory dish that takes less than an hour to make. The cooking is painless. Sauté onion and garlic in oil, then stir in tomato paste, cumin, and chili powder and cook a few minutes more to intensify flavor. Add broth, water, red lentils (which cook faster than their green or black counterparts), and diced carrot, and simmer for 30 minutes. Purée half the mixture and return it to the pot for a soup that strikes the balance between chunky and pleasingly smooth. A hint of lemon juice adds an up note that offsets the deep cumin and chili flavors. Featured in: *A Lentil Soup To Make You Stop, Taste And Savor.*

INGREDIENTS

- 3 Tbsp olive oil, more for drizzling
- 1 large onion, chopped
- 2 garlic cloves, minced
- 1 Tbsp tomato paste
- 1 tsp ground cumin
- ¼ tsp sea salt, more to taste
- ¼ tsp ground black pepper
- pinch of ground chili powder or cayenne, more to taste
- 1 quart chicken or vegetable broth
- 2 cups water
- 1 cup red lentils
- 1 large carrot, peeled and diced
- juice of ½ lemon, more to taste
- 3 Tbsp chopped fresh cilantro

***Three Bean Chili**
black, pinto, and kidney beans (we recommend making your beans from dried beans rather than from a can to avoid aluminum)
organic canned tomatoes
organic tomato sauce
garlic powder
cayenne pepper
chili powder
2 Tbsp quinoa, pre-cooked

***Stir Fry**
grapeseed oil
onions
garlic cloves
ginger powder
sea salt and pepper
2 kinds of mushrooms
zucchini
yellow squash
celery
red pepper and yellow pepper
    Serve on spaghetti squash as an option

***It's a stir fry kind of day**
grapeseed oil, garlic, onion, celery
a little bit of kale and a little bit of collard greens
zucchini, broccoli
spices: ginger, turmeric, cumin, onion powder, Mrs. Dash
    Always experimenting – we will probably have some quinoa with this.

Veggie Soup

Container of veggie broth, 1 white potato, 1 sweet potato, 1 cup cabbage, kale, a little parsley, several carrots, ½ a medium onion, couple stalks of celery, 2 cloves of garlic, 1 cup brown rice, ginger powder, sea salt, pepper, and turmeric to taste. Yum!

Chicken & Rice Soup

All organic:

chicken (2 pieces)

chicken broth

cayenne

curry

poultry seasoning

paprika

brown rice (cooked)

3 long carrots

2 baby sweet peppers

¼ onion (diced)

1 potato

2 garlic cloves

*Stir Fry

Servings: 4   Prep Time: 10 mins   Cook Time: 10 mins

2 cups chopped organic broccoli

2 cups chopped organic baby carrots

1 cup organic peas

1 cup organic pea pods

½ cup coconut aminos (soy sauce replacement)

1 - 2 Tbsp ginger

1 tsp pink salt

2 Tbsp coconut oil

SuperSmart Stir Fry Instructions:

Throw all ingredients into a frying pan and cook!

Yummy Stir Fry

snow peas, cauliflower, broccoli, asparagus, purple cabbage, onions, mushrooms, carrots, celery, garlic

Serve over brown rice

*Stir Fry

Serve over spaghetti squash or brown rice

mushrooms

zucchini

garlic

green beans

half an avocado

Sauce:

¼ cup grapeseed oil

Italian seasoning

cayenne pepper

* to make a spaghetti squash – heat in the oven for 30 minutes, remove, cut in half, deseed then bake at 375° for 45 - 60 minutes

Calories : 250 with squash, 380 with brown rice

*Vegetable Stir Fry

green beans

corn (be sure it is organic, non-GMO)

black beans

zucchini

broccoli

cayenne pepper

Himalayan salt

Serve over a half of a cooked spaghetti squash

Avocado Tomato Eggplant Rounds

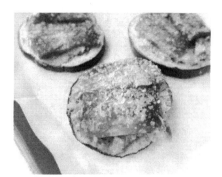

Prep Time: 5 mins   Cook Time: 20 mins   Total Time: 25 mins

Please use all organic ingredients when possible!

Author: Megan Lawson   Serves: 2

INGREDIENTS

- 1 small eggplant
- 1 avocado
- 1 tomato, sliced
- ½ tsp garlic powder
- ¼ tsp turmeric
- dash of cayenne pepper
- salt and pepper to taste

Instructions:

1. Preheat oven to 350°.
2. Cut eggplant into rounds. Place on baking sheet covered with parchment and bake for 20 min. Make sure to keep an eye after 12 minutes. Depending on size and oven heat, they could bake faster. They'll brown a little. You just don't want them to burn.
3. While they are baking, make the avocado mash using a fork to mix all of the seasonings and avocado together.
4. When the eggplants are done baking, allow to cool for at least 10 minutes.
5. Once cool, spread avocado mash, top with tomato and nutritional yeast.

Spicy African Yam Soup

sweet potatoes (2)

regular potatoes (2)

black beans (2 cans)

hot salsa

Sriracha sauce

garlic

zucchini (2)

brown rice

water

vegetable stock

Food Babe's Spaghetti Squash Casserole

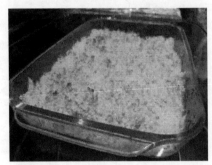

Prep Time: 1 hour   Cook Time: 35 mins   Total Time: 1 hour 35 mins

Serves: 6 - 8

INGREDIENTS

- 1 large spaghetti squash
- 1 cup dry quinoa
- 2 cups vegetable broth
- olive oil for spraying
- 1 ½ cups water
- 5 leaves fresh sage minced finely or ½ tsp dried
- ⅛ cup spelt or almond flour
- ½ tsp olive oil
- 3 cloves garlic, minced

157

- ¼ tsp sea salt
- ¼ tsp turmeric
- ¼ tsp red pepper flakes
- fresh ground pepper
- ⅓ cup nutritional yeast
- 1 Tbsp fresh lemon juice
- 1 tsp yellow mustard

Instructions:

Preheat oven to 350°.

Topping:

Make quinoa according to package instructions with vegetable broth instead of water

Spaghetti Squash:

Slice spaghetti squash in half and remove all seeds with spoon

Place spaghetti squash face down on large baking sheet, add ½ cup water and cover with foil

Bake spaghetti squash for 45 mins

Once baked, take a fork and scrape out inside of squash into a large baking dish

Cheese Sauce:

Combine water, flour, ground pepper, red pepper flakes, turmeric, and nutritional yeast and mix together to combine. Set aside

Heat a pan on medium heat, add olive oil and garlic

Sauté garlic for 2-3 mins, making sure not to burn

Add sage and cook lightly until fragrant

Next add the liquid, flour and spice mixture to the pan. The mixture should begin to bubble and start to thicken, if not – increase heat

Allow sauce to bubble for about 2 - 3 mins, and then add lemon juice and mustard and cook another 2 mins

Assembly of Casserole:

Pour cheese sauce evenly over squash in baking dish

Top with quinoa and lightly spray with olive oil

Bake at 350° for 20 - 25 mins and broil on high for last 5 - 10 mins to brown the top

Notes:

Makes approximately 6 - 8 servings. Great as a main dish or side dish for Thanksgiving! Also – this recipe can be made ahead and baked later (for 30 - 40 mins instead) – A huge time saver! *Cheese Sauce adapted from "Veganomican – The Ultimate Vegan Cookbook" ***Please buy all organic ingredients if possible***

Lentil Soup

Cook dried lentils as instructed on package. When about ¾ of the way done, add onion, celery, carrots, veggie broth, spices: sea salt, pepper, occasionally I add cumin and ginger powder. When finished add some fresh spinach and simmer until it is a bit wilted. Enjoy!

Cabbage Soup

INGREDIENTS

- 3-15oz cans fire-roasted tomatoes
- 3-15oz cans tomato sauce
- 2 cups quinoa (cooked separately)
- 2 packages pre-shredded cabbage
- 2 - 3 Tbsp Italian seasoning
- 1 Tbsp fresh garlic
- 1 Tbsp cayenne pepper
- water

Instructions:

Mix all ingredients in a crockpot and stir. Add water until it reaches the top of the cabbage. Let it simmer overnight. (Or cook on high for 2 hours.)

Notes:

Meat eaters – feel free to add ground beef or turkey that is hormone/antibiotic free instead of the quinoa (a pound fried up and added to all the ingredients).

For extra heat, add jalapeno peppers and/or some organic Sriracha sauce.

Lentil (or other bean) Burritos

Save some of the lentils you cooked for soup before adding the veggie broth and contents. Fry up the lentils in a pan with grapeseed, macadamia nut, or avocado oil with sea salt and pepper and a little onion. Once they are at a good consistency, add some organic salsa (mild, medium, hot). We also add a jalapeño (diced) to make it spicier.

Purchase soft spinach tortillas (my favorite) or Ezekiel tortillas for the "wrap" and vegan cheese made from cashews with a Mexican flavor or use a high quality dairy cheese (remember no hormones or antibiotics).

Place a scoop of lentil mixture in the center of the tortilla, pile on some vegan cheese, roll up and place in a dish that can be used for the oven.

Once you have filled all the wraps/tortillas, sprinkle with cheese you have saved for the top, and heat in the oven at 375° until the cheese melts. Enjoy with Beanito chips and salsa.

Vegetable and Bean Pot Pies with Potato Crust

Serves: 5

1 Tbsp extra virgin olive oil, divided

1 medium yellow onion, small diced

1 medium carrot, small diced

1 stalk celery, small diced

4 cloves garlic, minced

1 tsp minced fresh rosemary (about 1 sprig)

1 tsp tomato paste

1 medium zucchini, cut into ½ inch cubes

1 ½ cups cooked white beans, like navy or butter beans

salt and pepper, to taste

3 Tbsp whole spelt or almond flour

1 ½ cups vegetable stock

1 medium sweet potato or 6 to 7 mini new potatoes, thinly sliced, or a mixture

- Preheat oven to 375°. Place 5 ramekins or ovenproof dishes with 1 cup capacity on a baking sheet and set aside.

160

- Heat half the olive oil in large pot over medium heat. Add onions, carrots and celery, and sauté until onions are slightly softened, about 3 minutes. Add garlic, rosemary and tomato paste, and stir. Add zucchini and white beans to pot. Stir to combine. Season stew with salt and pepper.
- Sprinkle flour over vegetables and beans. Stir until flour is moistened and is starting to get slightly pasty. Pour in vegetable stock. Bring to a boil and then reduce to a simmer until slightly thickened, stirring occasionally, about 4 minutes.
- Divide stew among the 5 ramekins. Arrange sweet potato slices on top of ramekins in a fan or layered pattern. This will form your top crust. Gently brush the sweet potato slices with remaining oil. Season crusts with salt and pepper.
- Slide pot pies into the oven, and bake until the filling is bubbling and the sweet potato slices are tender and lightly browned on the edges, about 30 to 35 minutes.
- Serve pot pies hot.

** In each delicious serving: 217 Calories/ 8 g Protein/ 4 g Fat/ 39 g Carbs (4 g Sugar, 10 g Fiber) / 82 mg Sodium

Shaved Root Salad with Crispy Lentils
Serves: 6   Ready in 1 Hour

Dressing Ingredients:
2 Tbsp extra virgin olive oil
1 Tbsp pure maple syrup
1 Tbsp mustard
1 Tbsp filtered water
1 Tbsp apple cider vinegar
1 tsp prepared horseradish
1 clove garlic, grated
salt and pepper, to taste

<u>Salad</u>:

⅓ cup French or black beluga lentils, rinsed

½ tsp extra virgin olive oil

salt and pepper, to taste

2 small beets, peeled, or 1 medium

2 medium carrots, peeled

1 small celery root, peeled

2 Tbsp chopped fresh dill (about 2 sprigs), for garnish

- Preheat oven to 400°F
- <u>Make the dressing</u>: In jar with tight-fitting lid, combine olive oils, maple syrup, mustard, water, vinegar, horseradish, garlic, salt and pepper. Tightly secure lid, and shake jar vigorously until dressing has a creamy and smooth consistency. Set aside.
- <u>Make the salad</u>: Bring medium saucepan of water to a boil. Drop in lentils and a big pinch of salt. Bring to a boil again, and then reduce heat to a simmer until lentils are just tender, about 20 mins. Drain lentils and spread out on kitchen towel to dry.

  Transfer dried lentils to baking sheet. Toss lentils with olive oil, salt and pepper. Slide baking sheet into preheated oven, and roast until lentils have dried and browned slightly, about 8 mins. Remove from oven and set aside.

  Slice beets paper thin and place in large bowl. Slice carrots and add to bowl. Cut celery root down the middle lengthwise. Slice each half of celery root with the mandoline, and add slices to bowl.

  Season all sliced vegetables with salt and pepper, and toss.

  Toss sliced vegetables with 2/3 of the dressing. Transfer dressed vegetables to a serving platter. Scatter crispy lentils over vegetables. Pour remaining dressing over lentils. Garnish salad with fresh dill, and serve immediately.

**In each delicious serving: 89 Calories/ 1 g Protein/ 6 g Fat/ 8 g Carbs (4 g Sugar, 2 g Fiber) / 88 mg Sodium

Gingered Sweet Potato and Mung Bean Curry with Coconut

Serves: 5   Ready in 1 Hour

1 Tbsp virgin coconut oil

1 yellow onion, finely chopped

2 cloves garlic, minced

2-inch piece of fresh ginger peeled and minced

1 tsp ground cumin

½ tsp crushed red pepper flakes

¼ tsp ground cinnamon

¼ tsp ground turmeric

½ cup mung beans, rinsed

1 medium sweet potato, peeled and 1 inch diced

4 cups vegetable stock

14 oz can light coconut milk

1 tsp coconut aminos

3 cups baby spinach, lightly packed

½ cup cilantro leaves, roughly chopped

1 Tbsp fresh lime juice

sea salt and ground black pepper, to taste

- Heat coconut oil in large, heavy soup pot over medium heat. Add onions and sauté until lightly softened, about 3 minutes. Add garlic, ginger, cumin, red pepper flakes, cinnamon and turmeric to pot. Stir and cook until garlic is quite fragrant, about 30 secs. Add mung beans and sweet potato and stir to coat in the spices and onions. Pour vegetable stock into pot and stir again. Cover and bring stew to a boil. Then, reduce heat to a simmer. Cook stock, covered, until mung beans are just tender, about 25 mins.
- Pour coconut milk and coconut aminos into pot and stir. Bring stew to a boil once more. Add spinach, cilantro, lime juice, salt and pepper, and stir until spinach is wilted and bright green, about 2 mins. Check stew seasoning and adjust if necessary.

**In each delicious serving: 325 Calories/ 8 g Protein/ 10 g Fat/ 50 g Carbs (13 g Sugar, 10 g Fiber) / 362 mg Sodium

Lemony Whole Roasted Cauliflower

Serves: 4

1 head cauliflower, outer leaves trimmed

2 Tbsp extra virgin olive oil

zest and juice of 1 lemon

1 Tbsp Dijon mustard

¼ tsp sea salt

¼ cup chopped fresh parsley

- Preheat oven to 375°F
- Add cauliflower to glass or ceramic baking dish (cauliflower sizes fluctuate, so pick a dish that fits).
- In a small bowl, combine oil, lemon zest and juice, mustard and salt.
- Bake for 40 minutes to 1 hour, until cauliflower is tender when pierced with a knife (time dependent on size of cauliflower). Transfer to serving dish and sprinkle with parsley. Slice into wedges and serve.

**In each delicious serving: 118 Calories/ 4 g Protein/ 7 g Fat/ 12 g Carbs (5 g Sugar, 6 g Fiber) / 301 mg Sodium

"Creamy" Zucchini, Walnut and Thyme Soup

The "creamy" here comes from souped and blended walnuts. Use good quality nuts— they are important for taste as well as texture. I have written this up with walnuts and thyme, but I just know it would be fabulous with mint, basil and pine nuts.

Serves: 4

1 cup skin-on walnuts – toast for five minutes at 350°F

1 large onion, chopped

1 ½ Tbsp olive oil

1 ½ tsp dried thyme leaves (less if yours are quite strong-tasting)

2 bay leaves

4 garlic cloves, minced

6 cups chopped zucchini/summer squash – yellow or green

5 cups vegetable broth

zest of half a lemon (more to taste)

freshly ground pepper

fresh thyme leaves (lemon thyme if you have some) – optional dash of honey if needed, in case of slight bitterness

1. Heat the oil in a soup pot and add the onions. Sauté gently until translucent. Add the bay leaves, dried thyme and garlic, and sauté a few more minutes. When the garlic smells fragrant and the onions lose their raw smell, add the chopped zucchini and the walnuts. Stir and pour over the hot stock. Bring to a boil. Lower the heat to simmer and cook gently for 20 minutes, adding the lemon zest during the last minute or so.

2. Remove the pan from the heat and fish out the bay leaves. Ladle into a blender or use a hand-blender/immersion blender to blend the soup to a beautifully smooth texture. Test for seasoning and taste – adding pepper, salt and/or honey if need be. Add in the fresh thyme leaves, if using.

Kale Pesto

2 cups kale, packed, roughly chopped, stems removed

2 cloves garlic or more to taste

zest of 1 lemon

juice of 1 ½ lemons or more to taste

¼ cup raw almonds

½ cup extra virgin olive oil

¼ tsp sea salt or to taste

¼ tsp pepper or to taste

Place all ingredients in food processor on Low to reach desired texture.

*Serve Kale Pesto over zoodles – (zucchini noodles)

*Thanksgiving Cauliflower

If there's gravy involved, no one's gonna miss the potatoes.

Total Time: 1:45   Cook: 1:30   Serves: 6

INGREDIENTS

- 1 big head of cauliflower

- 4 Tbsp butter, melted (divided)
- 4 garlic cloves (skin-on)
- 6 sage leaves
- 4 sprigs fresh thyme
- 4 sprigs fresh rosemary
- sea salt
- freshly ground black pepper

Gravy:

- 1 Tbsp butter
- ½ onion, finely chopped
- 4 oz. cremini mushrooms, finely chopped
- 3 Tbsp unsalted butter
- 3 Tbsp almond flour
- 2 - 4 cups vegetable stock

Directions:

1. Preheat oven to 450°F

2. Rub the cauliflower all over with melted butter. Season with salt and pepper. Place in cast iron skillet, surrounded by garlic, 4 sage leaves, 2 sprigs of thyme and 2 sprigs of rosemary. Bake for 1 ½ hours until charred in parts and tender throughout, brushing with more melted butter through. Pierce the cauliflower with a paring knife skewer to check the tenderness.

3. Make gravy. Chop remaining thyme and rosemary leaves. Melt remaining butter in a small saucepan over medium heat. Add the onion and sauté until beginning to soften, about 3-5 minutes. Stir in the mushrooms and season mixture with salt and pepper. Add herbs and cook until the mushrooms are tender and browned. Add 1-2 cloves of the roasted garlic (skins removed), breaking up the cloves with a whisk or wooden spoon. Stir in flour and cook for 1 minute. Whisk in 2 cups of vegetable stock and bring mixture to a boil. Reduce heat slightly and simmer for 5 minutes, until the mixture has thickened to your desired consistency. Add more vegetable stock if desired.

Loaded Lentil Salad

Prep Time: 15 mins   Cook Time: 20 mins   Total Time: 35 mins

This hearty Loaded Lentil Salad is packed with protein, fiber, and warm veggies like roasted sweet potatoes, red onion, and Brussels sprouts. Perfect for a light lunch! Vegan and gluten-free.   Author: Alexis *sponsored by Hello Fresh* Serves: 4

INGREDIENTS

- 3 medium sweet potatoes, diced into ½ inch cubes
- 2 tsp Herbs de Provence
- 2 tsp pure maple syrup or honey
- ¼ cup extra virgin olive oil, divided
- 2 red onions, diced
- 16oz Brussels sprouts, thinly sliced
- 1 cup French lentils*
- 3 cups water
- ¼ cup balsamic vinegar
- ⅓ cup pepitas
- ½ tsp salt + pepper to taste

Instructions:

1. Preheat oven to 425°F. Line a baking sheet with foil or parchment paper.
2. Combine sweet potatoes, Herbs de Provence, maple syrup or honey, 1 Tbsp olive oil, and a pinch of salt in a medium boil. Spread onto prepared baking sheet and roast for about 11-13 minutes. Toss and roast until golden, another 11-13 minutes.
3. Heat ½ Tbsp olive oil in a medium pot over medium heat. Add onion and cook until softened, about 5 minutes. Add lentils and water. Bring to a boil then reduce heat to low and simmer until tender, about 15-20 minutes. Season with another pinch of salt and drain any excess water. Return to pot.
4. Heat ½ Tbsp olive oil in a medium pan over medium heat. Add Brussels sprouts and cook until golden brown, 4-5 minutes. Season with salt and pepper to taste.
5. Add balsamic vinegar and remaining 2 Tbsp olive oil to pot with lentils. Add Brussels sprouts, roasted sweet potatoes, and salt and pepper to taste. Top with pepitas and serve!

4 STEP VEGGIE BOWLS

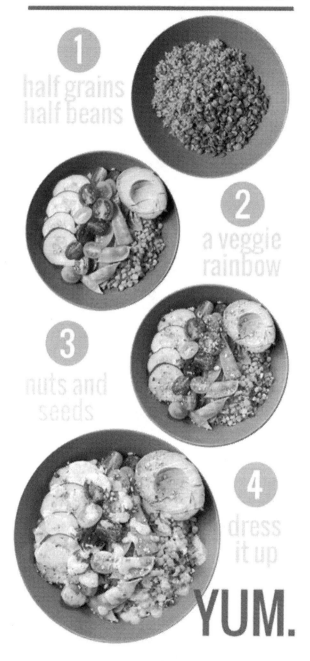

1 half grains half beans

2 a veggie rainbow

3 nuts and seeds

4 dress it up

YUM.

*Raw, Vegan Breakfast Pudding

Serves: 6-8

4 cups cashew milk

1 banana (ripe works best)

½ cup raw flaked oats (you can use organic rolled oats)

½ cup chia seeds

3 cups fresh fruit (strawberries, blueberries and raspberries)

1 tsp vanilla (optional)

pinch Himalayan sea salt (optional)

Instructions:

1. Blend banana into cashew milk.

2. Stir in the remaining ingredients.

3. Ladle into jars, cover and place in refrigerator overnight. Alternatively, you can just put in a glass bowl, cover and refrigerate overnight. It will be ready to go in the morning!

Oats are a great source of fiber. They also contain protein, thiamin, magnesium, phosphorus, zinc, manganese, selenium, and iron. They are filling and help prevent heart disease!* Chia seeds are high in omega 3's. Something that many of us are lacking. They also have fiber, protein, antioxidants and a wonderful filling quality, like the oats. And cashews are one of the healthiest nuts. They protect your heart and your bones, and studies have shown that a moderate amount of nuts can actually help you lower your risk of weight gain. If you don't like cashews, you can always substitute your favorite nut-milk.

Peanut Butter Chia Overnight Oats

Serves: 1

INGREDIENTS

¾ cup organic rolled oats

2 Tbsp chia seeds

½ tsp cinnamon

pinch of sea salt

1 cup unsweetened vanilla almond milk (or any plant milk)*

½ cup filtered water

1 tsp vanilla extract (optional)

1 ripe banana, mashed (but leave a few banana coins for topping!)

2 Tbsp organic peanut powder + 1 ½ Tbsp water (or any nut butter, to taste if not using powder)

1 - 2 Tbsp maple syrup, raw honey, or a few drops of liquid stevia for extra sweetness

Extras/Toppings:

cacao nibs (optional)

coconut flakes

crushed almonds or walnuts

sliced banana coins

extra sprinkles of cinnamon!

Instructions:

Add oats, chia seeds, cinnamon, and sea salt to a mason jar and mix well. Add in almond milk, water, vanilla, and mashed banana. Stir until combined.

In a small bowl, mix peanut powder with water until creamy. You can double the ingredients for extra peanut buttery flavor! Stir "peanut butter" mixture into mason jar. You can add toppings now or in the morning!

Refrigerate overnight or at least 4 hours. Dig in with a spoon and enjoy!

Notes:

* Other plant milk options: coconut milk, hemp milk, rice milk, flax milk, oat milk, cashew milk, etc.

** If overnight oats seem too dry for your liking in the morning, just add in a couple splashes of almond milk or water!

SIDE DISHES

*Easy salad
spinach

kale

strawberries

grapes

almonds

Dressing:

grapeseed oil

apple cider vinegar

fresh squeezed lemon juice or lemon oil (must be ingestible)

fresh squeezed orange juice or orange oil (must be ingestible)

Salad
spinach

kale (optional)

mushrooms

zucchini

half an avocado

berries (blueberries, raspberries, strawberries, whatever you like)

kiwi

mango

*for fewer calories you don't have to add so much fruit. Also, you can add nuts.

Dressing:

¼ cup grapeseed oil

¼ cup apple cider vinegar

lemon oil or juice

orange oil or juice

Mushrooms

INGREDIENTS

grapeseed oil

1 pound cultivated mushrooms, trimmed, halved or quartered

3 cloves garlic, peeled and crushed

salt and freshly ground black pepper

Directions:

Preheat oven to 450°. Lightly oil shallow baking pan large enough to hold mushrooms in single layer. Add mushrooms and toss with 2 to 3 Tbsp oil. Add garlic; season with salt; roast for 20 minutes, stirring on occasion; mushrooms should be browned. Season with pepper.

Quinoa Side Dish

Quinoa, garlic powder or several cloves sautéed, sweet potatoes cubed (cook briefly before cutting, it will make it easier), kale (you can buy frozen packets of these 3 ingredients together at Costco seasoned with garlic), add sliced or diced mushrooms, onion, cabbage, sea salt, pepper.

*Baked, Stuffed Acorn Squash

Cut an acorn squash in half (after it is baked) and add a little bit of olive oil and thyme. Top with a serving of brown rice and ¼ cup of walnuts

Sweet Potato Fries

Peel the sweet potatoes (1 or 2)

Cut into wedges

Put into a bowl and mix with ¼ cup grapeseed oil, cinnamon and sea salt or a combination of cayenne pepper and sea salt

Place on cooking tray

Sprinkle with more cinnamon or cayenne

Bake at 350° for 45-60 minutes

Sweet Potato Skins

Prep Time: 10 mins   Cook Time: 35 mins   Total Time: 45 mins

Serves: 8-10

INGREDIENTS

- 8 small sweet potatoes
- coconut oil
- 3 avocados, peeled and pitted
- 1 large tomato, diced
- ½ cup diced red onion
- ½ jalapeño, diced
- 1 lime, juiced
- ¼ cup chopped cilantro
- sea salt and pepper, to taste
- 1 cup cooked black beans
- 1 cup shredded vegan cheddar cheese

Instructions:

1. Preheat oven to 400°
2. Rub each sweet potato with coconut oil and place in the oven for 25-30 minutes or until fork tender.
3. While the sweet potatoes are cooking, in a bowl, make the guacamole. Start by mashing the avocado and then add the tomato, onion, jalapeño, lime juice, and cilantro. Season with salt and pepper to taste. Set aside.
4. When the sweet potatoes are done, take them out of the oven. Cut each one in half and scoop out half of the filling. Set the filling aside.
5. Sprinkle some of the black beans and cheese on each sweet potato half and place back in the oven to melt the cheese, 3-4 minutes.
6. When melted, take out of the oven and top with a scoop of guacamole. Enjoy!

Notes:

Please use all organic ingredients if possible Use leftover sweet potato filling as a side dish or freeze for later.

Salad with Chickpeas

Romaine lettuce, spinach, cucumbers, tomatoes, green onions, sea salt, extra virgin olive oil, ginger root, lemon (squeezed), vinegar, no-sugar dried raspberry, and chickpeas. Took me 15 minutes.

Cinnamon, Apple, Walnut, Kale and Quinoa Salad

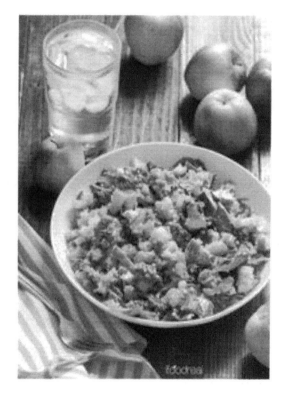

Author: Sara Wylie   Serves: 6

INGREDIENTS

- ⅔ cup dry or 2 cups cooked quinoa
- 3 large handfuls kale, stalks removed and finely chopped
- 3 medium apples, cored and diced (use sweet variety)
- 5 celery stalks, diced
- 1 cup walnut halves or pieces

Cinnamon Dressing:

- ¼ cup extra virgin olive oil
- ¼ cup apple cider vinegar
- 2 Tbsp maple syrup or honey
- ½ lemon (the juice)
- 1 tsp cinnamon
- 1 tsp salt
- ½ tsp ground black pepper

Instructions:

1. Cook dry quinoa according to package instructions. If using leftover quinoa, measure 2 cups. Add to a large mixing bowl along with kale, walnuts, apples and celery.
2. In a small skillet, toast walnuts on low-medium heat until lightly brown, about 5 minutes. Stir frequently and watch closely not to burn. Transfer to a bowl with other ingredients.
3. In a small bowl, whisk together Cinnamon Dressing ingredients, pour over salad and stir gently. Serve cold or warm, on its own or with chicken or turkey.

Notes/Storage Instructions:

Refrigerate salad without the dressing for up to 2 days. Dressing keeps well refrigerated for a few weeks. All dressed salad stays fresh in the fridge for up to 1 day.

Harvest Cobb Salad

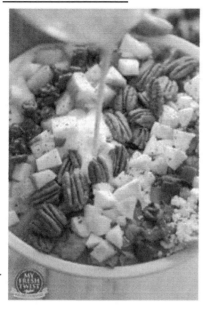

Total Time: 30 mins   Author: Sara Wylie   Serves: 4

INGREDIENTS

- 2 large eggs
- 6 cups chopped romaine lettuce
- 1 apple, diced
- 1 pear, diced
- ½ cup Pecan halves
- ⅓ cup dried cranberries
- ⅓ cup crumbled goat cheese
  Poppy Seed Dressing:
- ⅓ cup mayonnaise (or substitute)
- ¼ cup milk (or any plant milk option)
- 1 Tbsp raw honey
- 1 Tbsp apple cider vinegar
- 1 Tbsp poppy seeds

Instructions:

1. To make the poppy seed dressing, whisk together mayonnaise, milk, honey, apple cider vinegar and poppy seeds in a small bowl; set aside.

176

2. Place eggs in a large saucepan and cover with cold water by 1 inch. Bring to a boil and cook for 1 minute. Cover eggs with a tight-fitting lid and remove from heat; set aside for 8-10 minutes. Drain well and let cool before peeling and dicing.

3. To assemble the salad, place romaine lettuce in a large bowl; top with arranged rows of eggs, apple, pear, pecans, cranberries and goat cheese.

4. Serve immediately with poppy seed dressing.

Apple, Pecan and Feta Salad

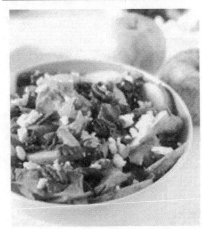

Prep Time: 15 mins   Total Time: 30 mins
Author: Sara Wylie   Serves: 1 big salad
INGREDIENTS

Salad:
- 3 cups kale, de-stemmed, washed and torn
- 1 apple, sliced thinly
- 2 Tbsp cranberries
- 2 Tbsp pecans
- 3 Tbsp feta cheese, crumbled

Honey-Apple Vinaigrette Dressing:
- 1 Tbsp honey
- 1 Tbsp apple cider vinegar
- 2 Tbsp olive oil
- ½ tsp salt

- ½ tsp ground black pepper

Instructions:

1. In a bowl, place the kale. Add the apples, cranberries, pecans and feta cheese on top – if you'd like, toss them in a bowl first then sprinkle on top.
2. Whisk the dressing together and pour over the salad.
3. Enjoy!

Sweet and Salty Fall Harvest Salad

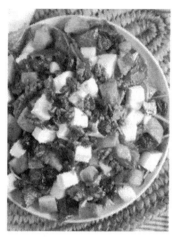

Prep Time: 1 hour

Author: Sara Wylie   Serves: 4

INGREDIENTS

Salad:

- 1 large butternut squash, peeled, seeded and cubed
- 3 Tbsp extra virgin olive oil, divided
- sea salt and freshly ground black pepper
- ½ cup chopped pecans
- 1 Tbsp unsalted butter
- at least 2 Tbsp of chosen sweetener (or brown sugar substitute)
- 1 bunch of kale, washed, stems removed, and roughly chopped (about 8 cups)
- 6 oz brie, cubed
- 1 large apple, cored and roughly chopped

- ½ cup dried cranberries
  <u>For the maple vinaigrette</u>:
- 2 Tbsp pure maple syrup
- up to ⅓ cup extra virgin olive oil
- 1 tsp Dijon mustard (or substitute)
- 1 Tbsp apple cider vinegar
- ¾ tsp sea salt

Instructions:

1. Preheat oven to 425°F. Spread the squash out on a large baking sheet and drizzle with 2 Tbsp of olive oil, then sprinkle with some salt and pepper. Roast for 35 minutes, toss the squash and roast for another 15 to 20 minutes, tossing periodically until the squash is browned and softened.

2. While the squash roasts, make the candied pecan clusters. Ready a Silpat or line a baking sheet with parchment paper; set aside. Heat the butter and brown sugar substitute over medium heat in a medium nonstick pan until bubbling. Toss the pecans into the butter-sugar mixture until coated. Cook, stirring occasionally, until the sugar liquefies and turns a dark amber color. Pour the pecans out onto the Silpat or parchment paper and spread them out with a rubber spatula. Allow them to cool completely before breaking them up into clusters.

3. Make the vinaigrette: Whisk the maple syrup, ¼ cup olive oil, mustard, vinegar and salt together in a medium bowl or shake it all together in a mason jar. Whisk in additional olive oil in small increments up to ⅓ cup total until you reach your desired dressing consistency.

4. In a large bowl, toss the kale with the remaining 1 Tbsp of olive oil. Massage the oil into the kale with your hands until the kale turns bright green and glossy, about 2-3 minutes.

5. Top the kale with the squash, brie, apples, cranberries and pecan clusters. Drizzle the maple vinaigrette over the top of the salad before serving while the squash is still warm.

Roasted Brussel Sprouts

INGREDIENTS

1 ½ pounds Brussels sprouts, ends trimmed and yellow leaves removed

1 tsp sea salt

½ tsp freshly ground black pepper

3 Tbsp coconut oil, or melted ghee

Instructions:

Preheat oven to 400°F

In a large resealable plastic bag, place all of your ingredients inside and seal the bag, then shake well to coat the Brussels sprouts. Pour the contents out onto a baking sheet and insert them into the oven.

Bake for 30-45 minutes, while shaking the pan every 5-7 minutes (this is for browning). If they start to burn, reduce the heat. The Brussels sprouts will come out dark brown, almost black, when they are fully cooked. Serve as soon as you pull them out of the oven. You can add more pepper or salt if needed for seasoning...or really spice them up like I have with some cayenne pepper and other spices!!

Cucumber Salad Recipe

INGREDIENTS

4 medium cucumbers, seedless if desired

1 Tbsp sea salt

1 oz of minced onion

¼ cup of chopped fresh dill

3 - 4 oz of Vegenaise

¼ tsp black pepper

juice of one lemon

Method:

1. Trim off ends of cucumbers and peel alternate stripes on them (or peel completely, or just leave the peel on like I do).

2. Slice thin and toss in bowl with salt; allow to cure for 10-12 minutes.

3. Rinse off salt thoroughly, allow to drain.

4. Add onion, dill and black pepper, then add lemon juice (more can be added if desired)

5. Add Vegenaise and adjust creaminess as desired.

Chickpea Salad

Prep Time: 10 minutes   Total Time: 10 minutes

Servings: 6   Author: Holly N.

INGREDIENTS

- 1 avocado
- ½ fresh lemon
- 1 can chickpeas , drained (19 oz)
- ¼ cup sliced red onion
- 2 cups grape tomatoes , sliced
- 2 cups diced cucumber
- ½ cup fresh parsley
- ¾ cup diced green bell pepper

Dressing:

- ¼ cup olive oil
- 2 Tbsp apple cider vinegar
- ½ tsp cumin
- Italian spice mix
- salt and pepper

Instructions:

1. Cut avocado into cubes and place in bowl. Squeeze the juice from ½ lemon over the avocado and gently stir to combine.
2. Add remaining salad ingredients and gently toss to combine.
3. Refrigerate at least one hour before serving.

Variations: Add cooked black beans, maybe some cilantro, onions

Balsamic Drizzled Brussels Sprouts

If you're looking for an appetizing way to prepare Brussels sprouts, look no further than this Balsamic Drizzled Brussels Sprouts recipe from *Naturally Savvy*. The balsamic vinegar adds that much needed flavor to the Brussels sprouts, and in no time your family and friends might be back for seconds.

INGREDIENTS

- 2 pounds Brussels sprouts, trimmed and halved
- 2 Tbsp coconut oil
- 2 cloves garlic, finely chopped
- large pinch of Himalayan salt
- freshly ground black pepper
- 1 to 2 Tbsp balsamic vinegar (add more or less to taste)

Procedure:

1. Heat oven to 400°F. On a large rimmed baking sheet or in a large casserole dish, toss the Brussels sprouts with oil, garlic, salt and a few grinds of freshly ground pepper.
2. Roast until tender and slightly golden, approximately 25 minutes.
3. Remove from the oven and drizzle with 1 to 2 Tbsp (or more) of balsamic vinegar. Taste and adjust seasoning if necessary.

This recipe makes six to eight servings.

Quinoa Tabouli

I like to divide this into ½ cup - 1 cup portions. Excellent for Food Prepping or Lunches on-the-go as it's delicious served cold or at room temperature.

3 cups cooked quinoa

4 - 5 small tomatoes diced

1 small red onion diced

3 - 4 medium cucumbers peeled and diced

1 cup roughly chopped fresh parsley

juice from 3 - 4 fresh lemons

1 – 1 ½ Tbsp avocado oil or extra virgin olive oil to taste

sea salt, black pepper

Place everything in a large bowl and combine. Adjust seasoning, lemon juice, and olive oil to taste.

Fall Harvest Salad with Maple Vinaigrette

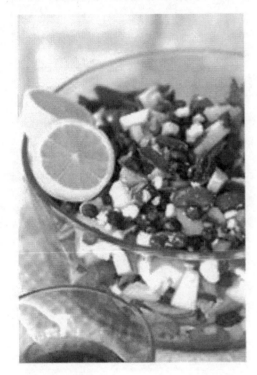

INGREDIENTS

- 1 (14-ounce) can kidney beans, drained, rinsed
- ½ pomegranate, arils removed
- 6 ounces goat cheese, crumbled
- 2 Granny Smith apples, diced
- 4 celery stalks, diced
- ½ red onion, diced
- 2 cups spinach, chopped
- ¾ cup pecans, toasted
- ¾ cup raisins
- 1 cucumber, peeled, diced

For the maple vinaigrette:

- ¼ cup olive oil
- ½ Tbsp balsamic vinegar
- 2 Tbsp maple syrup
- 1 tsp lemon juice
- salt, to taste
- pepper, to taste

Instructions:

1. In a large bowl, toss together all salad ingredients.
2. In a separate bowl, whisk together vinaigrette ingredients. Taste and adjust to your liking (add more maple syrup for additional sweetness).
3. Chill each separately in the fridge. Drizzle vinaigrette over salad just before serving.

Sesame Kale Salad

Serves: 3   Prep Time: 5 min   Cook Time: 15 min   Total Time: 20 min

INGREDIENTS

1 cup quinoa

1 Tbsp coconut oil/sesame oil

½ of a red onion

1 clove garlic, minced

3 cups kale, de-stemmed and torn

2 cups broccoli florets (about 1 small head)

2 Tbsp coconut aminos (similar to soy sauce)

2 Tbsp water

juice from ½ - 1 lime, depending on your liking

½ Tbsp Dijon mustard

1 tsp fresh ginger, minced (or powdered)

½ tsp black pepper

dash of red pepper flakes (optional)

2 Tbsp sesame seeds (black or white) – you could also use any other seed you like

Instructions:

Combine 1 cup quinoa with 2 cups water in a medium-sized pot. Bring to a boil and reduce heat to simmer for about 15 minutes or until all water has been absorbed. Meanwhile, in a small saucepan, melt the coconut oil on medium-high heat. Add the red onion and sauté for 2-3 minutes. Add the garlic, kale, broccoli. Sauté for about 3 minutes.

In a small bowl, combine the water, lime juice, Dijon mustard, ginger, pepper, red pepper flakes and seeds. Add mixture to saucepan with vegetables and mix until well combined. Cook for about 2 more minutes.

Once quinoa is finished cooking, scoop it into 2-3 bowls and top with the vegetable mixture. Add extra coconut aminos as needed.

Salad Dressing

This is a great and easy salad dressing for Mexican inspired dishes. Great on tacos and burritos too!

Servings: 10

INGREDIENTS

> ½ avocado
> ½ cup unsweetened nut milk
> ¼ tsp minced garlic
> ¼ tsp sea salt
> ¼ tsp fresh ground black pepper
> ¼ tsp chili powder
> juice of one wedge of lime

Directions:

Place all ingredients in a food processor or blender and pulse until everything is creamy.

Makes about 10 Tablespoons of dressing.

Serving Size: 1 Tablespoon

Recipe submitted by SparkPeople user KIMBERLEIGH06.

Quinoa Salad

Cook Quinoa then cool. Dice up some cucumber, tomato, zucchini, onion, celery, cilantro and add to quinoa.

Dressing: olive oil, Italian spice, apple cider vinegar

DESSERTS

Chocolate Fondue

Blend together:

coconut oil

cacao powder

almond milk

almond butter

Dip pieces of yellow honeydew into blended mixture!

Spiced Pumpkin Freezer Fudge

Total time: 2 hrs 10 mins   Cook Time: 2 hrs   Prep Time: 10 mins

Serves: 18 bars   Recipe by: Megan Olson

This no-bake pumpkin fudge is made with only six wholesome ingredients and absolutely no processed sugar.

Tools:

10x5 baking pan

Parchment Paper

Mixing Bowl

Spatula

INGREDIENTS

½ cup coconut butter

¼ cup maple syrup

½ tsp vanilla extract

¾ cup organic pumpkin purée

2 Tbsp coconut flour

2 tsp pumpkin spice

Instructions:

Line a baking sheet with parchment paper. Set aside.

In a mixing bowl, mix together the coconut butter, maple syrup and vanilla until smooth.

Add the remaining ingredients and mix until combined. Do not over mix. If the batter is too stiff, add ¼ cup coconut oil and stir until smooth.

Transfer the batter to the prepared baking sheet and spread into a smooth layer.

Place in the freezer for 2 hours or until frozen.

Slice into 18 bars and serve. Keep the leftover bars in the freezer.

Nudge (not fudge)

INGREDIENTS (I usually double the recipe)

6 Tbsp organic nut butter*

3 Tbsp coconut oil

3 Tbsp raw honey

2 Tbsp cocoa or cacao powder

½ tsp concentrated natural vanilla extract

pinch of sea salt

½ cup walnuts or cashews crushed (I placed them in a Ziplock bag and crushed them)

METHOD:

Place all ingredients except for the cashews/walnuts into a medium sized bowl and mix until well combined and looking deliciously chocolatey. Stir in the nuts. Pour the mixture into a silicone loaf tin, or glass container, or plastic if you must. Place in the fridge to set – or even the freezer with a lid on it. Slice and serve. It only takes a couple of hours to set. However, the longer you leave it the firmer it will become. I like it best the day after making.

Store in the fridge as it will melt at room temperature.

Enjoy knowing you aren't feeding the kids or yourself nasty refined sugars.

*You can use organic peanut butter or almond butter or any nut butter or... if you prefer, use organic peanut butter powder like I did. STAY AWAY FROM PB2 – To use the organic powdered peanuts, you will need to add water to create your butter and then measure it out for the recipe.

Chocolate Orange Chia Seed Pudding

CAUTION: You will want to eat more than 1 serving...I did and so did Mike!!!

Total Time: 2 minutes   Servings: 8

Per Serving: 109 calories   Fat 4 g   Carbs 17 g   Protein 3 g

INGREDIENTS

1 ½ cups almond milk (or other non-dairy milk)

⅓ cup (2 oz.) chia seeds

5 drops Young Living orange essential oil

½ tsp cinnamon

½ tsp vanilla

3 Tbsp raw cacao powder

~5 pitted dates soaked in hot water, then drained

Instructions:

Place all ingredients into blender, like a Vitamix.

Assemble pudding as desired. I just put it in a container and refrigerate for a couple of hours.

Notes/Nutritional Benefits:

• Nothing refined, made with whole food sweetener – dates: Dates are a great source of potassium, fiber, and a source of magnesium, making them great for heart health. The added fiber, helps to lessen blood sugar spikes and moderate blood sugar.

• Great source of fiber, 8.5 g, important for blood sugar regulation, satiety, reducing blood pressure, and boosting digestive health.

• High in plant-based calcium, 27% DV, shown to be better absorbed by the body than animal source, it's important for bone and dental health.

• Good source of plant-based iron, 10% DV, important for oxygenation of blood.

• Good source of plant-based protein, 4.3 g, important for tissue repair.

Protein Packed Cookies – by Dr. Jockers

½ cup of sunflower seeds

½ cup of high-quality protein powder

¼ cup of honey

1 tsp of vanilla

1 tsp of cinnamon

2 Tbsp of coconut oil

1/8 cup of water

Instructions:

Preheat oven to 300°F

Roughly chop sunflower seeds (or other nuts you may wish to use) in the blender until broken up into chunks.

Place all ingredients into a bowl and stir together. If you notice that it is too crumbly, then try adding in another tablespoon of coconut oil and possibly more water.

Scoop cookies onto a cookie tray.

Gently press the cookies down to flatten.

Makes about 18 cookies.

Bake for about 15 minutes.

Additional Notes:

You can use 2 cups coconut shreds if you do not have/want sunflower seeds.

You can use any other kind of nut or seed.

You can use any flavored or unflavored protein powder to change up the flavor.

You can put the coconut whipped cream recipe (https://drjockers.com/coconut-whipped-cream/) in between to make an incredible coconut cookie sandwich!

Dr. Jockers Comments:

This is a fun and tasty recipe that is full of fiber, healthy fats and clean protein. It is low carb, ketogenic and helps us to stabilize our blood sugar and burn fat.

If you are following an autoimmune nutrition plan, then you may want to avoid the sunflower seeds and instead use extra coconut flakes. Coconut flakes are a great source of medium chain fats that help us to burn fat and provide immediate fuel for our body and brain. They also provide good fiber for our microbiome.

Stevia is my preferred sweetener because it is one hundred times sweeter than sugar and has no effect on our blood sugar.

You can use a wide variety of protein powders, such as grass-fed whey protein that is full of branched chain amino acids to help support the development of lean body mass.

Healthy Four Ingredient Breakfast Brownies

Protein packed brownies which are perfectly acceptable for breakfast and need just four ingredients! Moist, soft and gooey on the inside yet tender on the outside, these flourless breakfast brownies are vegan, gluten free, paleo and refined-sugar free!

INGREDIENTS

3 medium, overripe bananas OR 1 cup mashed sweet potato OR 1 cup mashed pumpkin OR mix of all 3

½ cup smooth nut butter or almond butter (can sub for any nut/seed butter)

2 Tbsp - ¼ cup cocoa or cacao powder (more = richer taste)

1 - 2 scoops of protein powder

handful of chocolate chips, optional (cocoa or cacao nibs or carob)

Instructions:

Preheat oven to 350°, grease a small cake pan or loaf pan with coconut oil and set aside.

In a small pan on stovetop, melt your nut butter.

In a blender, food processor, or using your hands, combine the mashed mixture, cocoa or cacao powder, protein powder and nut butter until smooth.

Pour the mixture into the greased pan, top with optional chocolate chips and bake for around 20 minutes or until baked through. Remove from the oven and allow to cool completely before slicing into pieces.

Notes:

You don't need to blend or process all ingredients, but doing so lends a smoother texture – although I do like my banana chunks in them.

These brownies are not super sweet, it depends on the protein powder you choose and how sweet it is. Adjust accordingly if you'd like a very sweet brownie by adding a little stevia or honey perhaps.

Brownies are best kept and enjoyed refrigerated. They are also freezer friendly.

My (Lillian's) edited version from Arman @ thebigmansworld

Sweet Potato Brownies

MY VERSION: INGREDIENTS

1 cup mashed sweet potato

½ cup smooth nut butter of choice (I recommend almond or cashew butter – or the organic peanut powder from Costco – add water)

2 Tbsp maple syrup or raw honey

¼ cup cocoa or cacao powder

handful of carob chips (optional)

Directions:

Preheat oven to 350°F and grease a small cake/loaf pan.

On the stove, melt nut butter with maple syrup/honey.

In a large bowl add the mashed sweet potato, melted nut butter, maple syrup, and cocoa or cacao powder and mix well.

Fold in carob chips.

Pour mixture into greased pan and bake for 20 minutes or until baked through. Remove from the oven and allow to cool completely before slicing and refrigerating. These brownies are best when cooled completely. Store in fridge or freezer and ENJOY!

Incredible Apple Carrot Quinoa Balls

1 cup (loosely packed) coarsely grated carrots (about 2 medium)

½ cup (packed) coarsely grated peeled apple (about 1 Gala or Fuji works well)

½ cup quinoa flakes

⅓ cup creamy unsweetened sunflower seed butter (I used organic Sunbutter)

3 - 4 Tbsp pure maple syrup

1 Tbsp ground chia seeds

1 tsp ground cinnamon

¼ tsp baking soda

¼ tsp Celtic sea salt or Himalayan salt

¼ cup raisins or dried currants

Preheat oven to 350°F, and line a baking sheet with parchment paper.

Grate the carrot in your food processor, and hand grate the apple for the best results.

In a large bowl, combine the carrot and apple with the dry ingredients, and then mix in the sunflower seed butter and maple syrup.

Stir to combine thoroughly and form a cohesive mass of dough. Then mix in the raisins.

Using moist hands, roll tablespoons of the dough into balls and place them 1-2 inches apart on the lined baking sheet.

Bake the balls for about 20 minutes.

Cool completely, and store in an airtight container in the fridge.

Makes about 18 moist and chewy balls.

published by Pure Living Press Hallie Klecker at Daily Bites.

No Bake Cookies

½ cup raw honey

2 Tbsp cocoa or cacao (reg. or dark)

¼ cup coconut milk (or almond milk)

¼ cup coconut oil

½ tsp vanilla

¼ cup almond butter (cashew, sunflower, organic peanut butter)

1 ½ - 1 ¾ cup quick oats

Combine first five ingredients in saucepan. Bring to boil and cook 2 ½-3 min. Turn off heat and stir in almond butter till smooth, then add quick oats and stir till coated. Drop by teaspoonfuls onto parchment paper. Let cool. It may help the firmness to refrigerate them for at least 30 min.

**add some unsweetened coconut along with the oats for variety & some chia seeds for binding a bit better... or... add more nut butter and limit the cocoa or cacao and they taste more like peanut butter cookies.

Ice Cream

INGREDIENTS

Serves 4 people

- 2 large cans of organic full-fat coconut milk
- 1 frozen banana
- 4 large dates, pitted
- 1 - 2 tsp vanilla extract
- pinch of cinnamon

METHOD:

1. Put the cans of coconut milk in the fridge to chill overnight. In the morning flip the cans over, open them and pour the liquid at the top of the can into a separate bowl.
2. Scrape the remaining coconut milk fat into a blender as this is the good stuff that we'll use for the recipe.
3. Now combine all of the ingredients into a high-speed blender/food processor and blend until you have a nice thick and creamy consistency. After blending all the ingredients, pour the goodness into a freezer-safe container and give it a good stir every half hour or so to avoid it becoming too solid. You may have to do this 3 or 4 times but it's well worth it.

Berry Coconut Milk Ice Cream

INGREDIENTS

1 can of full fat coconut milk

½ tsp vanilla extract

1 full cup frozen organic berries of choice

pinch of sea salt

¼ tsp stevia

Optional Ingredients:

1 scoop of vanilla protein

Berry Coconut Milk Ice Cream Instructions:

Blend coconut milk, sweetener, salt, vanilla, and berries until smooth.

Place a sheet of parchment paper on deep baking dish. Pour the coconut milk onto the parchment paper and then freeze for several hours, until hard.

Once frozen, pull the coconut milk off the parchment paper and break into chunks.

Add coconut mixture to the blender.

Process until smooth, scooping down the sides as necessary.

Snowball Cookies

1 cup almond butter (cashew, organic peanut butter)

2 Tbsp raw honey

½ cup carob powder (or cacao or cocoa)

2 tsp cinnamon

1 tsp nutmeg

2 pinches sea salt

½ cup dried shredded coconut

Directions:

Combine all ingredients except coconut in a large bowl and mix thoroughly.

Form into balls and roll in coconut flakes.

Chocolate Chip Cookies

INGREDIENTS

3 cups pecans OR walnuts (soaked overnight, drained, and allowed to air dry)

12 Medjool dates, pitted

1 tsp orange zest

1 tsp cinnamon

½ tsp Celtic or Himalayan sea salt (or to taste)

1 ½ Tbsp raw coconut oil (best if soft but not liquid)

3 Tbsp carob chips or cacao nibs

Option: Balls may be rolled in unsweetened coconut or chopped nuts.

Instructions:

1. Place dates in food processor with "S" blade and process until smooth.

2. Add walnuts (or pecans), cinnamon, salt, and coconut oil. Process until well blended.

3. Add carob chips and blend just until chips are well distributed.

4. Remove from processor and form tablespoons of mix into balls.

5. Then flatten into round cookies or leave in ball form.

6. Refrigerate till time to serve. ENJOY!

Pumpkin Nut Butter Brownies

Servings: 6-8

1 ½ cups pumpkin puree

¾ cup nut butter

¼ cup raw cacao powder

5 dates, pitted

2 cups dark chocolate, melted (at least 60% cacao)

1 cup canned coconut milk

Instructions:

1. Preheat oven the 350°, and grease a baking pan lightly with coconut oil.

2. Add the pumpkin puree, nut butter, cocoa or cacao powder and dates to a high speed blender or food processor. Pulse just until a thick batter is formed.

3. Pour the mixture into the greased pan and bake for 15-20 minutes, or until a toothpick comes out clean from the center. (Could take up to 20-30 minutes. Put them back in the oven for 5 minutes at a time until done.)

4. Remove from the oven and allow to cool in the pan completely.

5. In a small bowl mix the melted chocolate with coconut milk. Whisk until well combined.

6. Pour the chocolate mixture on top of the brownie and level it with a spatula. Refrigerate for 3 hours (or overnight)

Modified Recipe is from Clean Food Crush

4 Ingredient Ice Cream

INGREDIENTS

• 2 bananas, cut into 1-inch slices (frozen)

• ½ cup frozen strawberries, sliced

- 2 Tbsp almond milk
- ½ tsp vanilla

Instructions:

1. Place banana slices on a plate, separating each slice. Place slices in freezer for 2 hours (overnight is best!).

2. Remove strawberries and bananas from freezer and place in food processor, blend until they are the consistency of soft serve ice cream.

3. Add almond milk (more or less for desired texture) and vanilla and blend until smooth and well-mixed.

4. Transfer ice cream to a freezer container and freeze until solid. (Don't have to wait if fruit is frozen, it is like soft serve ice cream.)

5. Scoop with ice cream scoop and serve.

Matcha Pistachio Bliss Balls

INGREDIENTS

¾ cup raw cashews

¼ cup raw pistachios, shelled

6 Medjool dates, pitted

¼ cup shredded coconut, unsweetened

2 tsp matcha powder

1 Tbsp coconut oil

¼ cup pistachios, chopped (for rolling)

Instructions:

Place all the ingredients (except the last ¼ cup pistachios) into a food processor. Process for one minute or until finely chopped and blended.

Using an ice cream scoop or tablespoon, scoop out balls of mixture. Roll between your hands to create evenly sized balls.

When all balls have been rolled, roll them again through the chopped pistachios and press firmly into the balls.

Refrigerate for 15 minutes then enjoy.

You can really use any frozen fruit to make this.

SNACKS

Extra Green Guacamole

INGREDIENTS

1 cup of cooked and cooled (or jarred) organic chickpeas

1 organic lemon, juiced

as much or as little organic cilantro as you like (I usually use about a small handful)

2 tsp organic extra virgin olive oil

½ avocado

pink Himalayan salt and pepper to taste

I sometimes spice this up with half of an organic jalapeño, with the seeds removed.

Directions:

You can prepare this dip one of two ways. You can mix the ingredients together by hand in a bowl, or if you want a smoother and creamier consistency, you can chuck everything in a blender for about a minute until everything is combined.

Chia Protein Bites

INGREDIENTS

2 Tbsp almond butter

2 ½ Tbsp raw honey

1 Tbsp coconut oil

1 scoop of high quality protein powder

5 Tbsp raw cacao powder

pinch of Himalayan pink salt

1 - 2 Tbsp chia seeds

Instructions:

1. Gather ingredients and place into a blender or a bowl.
2. Blend or mix by hand until smooth.
3. Batter will be a little sticky and oily.
4. Scoop batter into bite size balls/cookies and place onto a non-stick surface.
5. Eat right away or store in refrigerator.

Vegan Spinach Dip

Prep Time: 15 mins   Cook Time: 35 mins   Total Time: 50 mins

Rich, creamy, warm and cheesy Vegan Spinach Dip that makes the perfect appetizer.

Author: Ceara

Serves: 2 heaping cups

INGREDIENTS

½ cup cashews, soaked

1 medium white onion, diced

½ cup frozen spinach (measured after defrosting)

¼ cup aquafaba (liquid from the chickpea can)

2 cups cooked or canned chickpeas

2 - 3 Tbsp nutritional yeast

1 Tbsp tahini

1 tsp apple cider vinegar

2 - 3 splashes hot sauce

1 ½ tsp garlic powder

2 tsp onion powder

¼ tsp paprika

1 tsp sea salt (or to taste)

pinch black pepper

chili powder (for garnish, optional)

Directions:

Soak ½ cup cashews overnight or in boiling water for 20 minutes.

Preheat oven to 375°F

Over medium-high heat, sauté diced onion in a splash of water (or dollop of oil) for 5 minutes until translucent.

Allow frozen spinach to defrost (or microwave on low for 30-second increments) and measure out ½ lightly packed cup of defrosted spinach, pressing out some of the water in the measuring cup.

Add soaked cashews, sautéed onion and aquafaba to a high-speed blender (like a Vitamix) and blend until creamy smooth.

Add chickpeas, defrosted spinach, nutritional yeast, tahini, apple cider vinegar, hot sauce and spices (garlic and onion powder, paprika, sea salt and pepper) to the blender. Using the tamper, blend for several pulses until the chickpeas are just creamy and still a little bit chunky. If you do not have a high-powered blender, pulse and scrape down the sides so your spices are evenly distributed when blending.

Transfer to an oven safe dish and bake for 30 to 35 minutes until the tip of the dip is crispy. Sprinkle with a pinch of chili powder before serving.

Notes:

If you do not have aquafaba on hand, use water or vegetable broth. You may have to adjust the spices and salt a bit to taste if you use water.

Easy Smooth Hummus

Prep Time: 10 minutes

Why we love this recipe. When we first figured out how to make our own hummus, we were shocked at how easy (and fast) it is. With just a few simple tricks, you really can make creamy smooth hummus at home and yes, we really do think it's better than store-bought.

What you need to know. Two things here. First, we use canned chickpeas, which is much, much quicker than using dried. Some swear by soaking and cooking their own dried chickpeas, but we're just not that organized and love that canned chickpeas means we can enjoy our hummus in 10 minutes. Second, our recipe calls for tahini, a creamy paste made from sesame seeds. You can usually find tahini in larger grocery stores or specialty markets.

Equipment you'll need. A mesh strainer or colander, food processor, silicone spatula, measuring cups and spoons.

Yield: Makes about 1 ½ cups or enough for 4 to 6 snack portions

INGREDIENTS

- One 15-ounce can (425 grams) chickpeas, also called garbanzo beans
- ¼ cup (59 ml) fresh lemon juice, about 1 large lemon

- ¼ cup (59 ml) tahini, we use Krinos or homemade tahini (it's easy to make)
- half of a large garlic clove, minced
- 2 Tbsp extra virgin olive oil, plus more for serving
- ½ to 1 tsp kosher salt, depending on taste
- ½ tsp ground cumin
- 2 - 3 Tbsp water
- dash of ground paprika for serving

Directions:

Preparing the Hummus

- In the bowl of a food processor, combine tahini and lemon juice. Process for 1 minute. Scrape sides and bottom of bowl, then turn on and process for 30 seconds. This extra time helps "whip" or "cream" the tahini, making smooth and creamy hummus possible.
- Add the olive oil, minced garlic, cumin and the salt to the whipped tahini and lemon juice mixture. Process for 30 seconds, scrape sides and bottom of bowl, then process another 30 seconds.

Adding the Chickpeas

- Open can of chickpeas, drain liquid then rinse well with water. Add half of the chickpeas to the food processor, then process for 1 minute. Scrape sides and bottom of bowl, add remaining chickpeas and process for 1 to 2 minutes or until thick and quite smooth.

Creating the Perfect Consistency

- Most likely the hummus will be too thick or still have tiny bits of chickpea. To fix this, with the food processor turned on, slowly add 2 - 3 Tablespoons of water until the consistency is perfect.

Baked Kale Chips Recipe (My Favorite)

INGREDIENTS

- 2 bunches kale
- 2 heaping Tbsp almond butter (or any savory nut butter)
- 1 Tbsp extra virgin olive oil
- ½ tsp ground cumin

- ½ tsp chili powder (or substitute curry powder, we make them both ways)
- ½ tsp garlic powder
- 1/8 tsp cayenne pepper
- ½ tsp salt

Directions:

1. Preheat oven to 350°F. Wash the kale and dry thoroughly with paper towels. Pull the leaves off the center ribs in large pieces, and pile on a baking sheet. Discard the ribs.

2. In a small bowl mix the nut butter, oil, spices, and salt. Pour over the kale. Use your hands to massage the kale leaves until each one is evenly coated with the spice mixture. You don't want any of the leaves to be drenched in the mixture, so take your time doing this. The more evenly the kale leaves are coated, the better they will bake.

3. Lay the kale leaves out flat on 3-4 full sized baking sheets (work in batches if necessary.) Do not overlap. Bake for 10-11 minutes until crisp, but still green. Cool for a few minutes on the baking sheet before moving. If some kale chips are still a little flimsy or damp, remove the crisp chips and place the damp chips back in the oven for a few more minutes. Store in an air-tight container.

Kale Chips

kale, rinsed and dried
1 Tbsp olive oil
2 Tbsp white balsamic vinegar
¼ tsp sea salt

Preheat oven to 350°F. Remove kale from the stems and tear into bite size pieces. Save the stems for juicing. Lay kale pieces on a lined or greased baking sheet. In a small bowl, mix oil, vinegar and salt. With a silicone brush, gently brush mixture onto the kale pieces. Bake in the oven for about 10 minutes or until pieces become crispy. They are so good, I eat the whole tray as soon as they come out! Enjoy! ☺

Cinnamon Red Hots Tea

By the cup:

one green tea bag—I like the Kirklands green tea with matcha powder

1 small cinnamon stick (3-4 inches)

1/16th tsp cayenne pepper

(I typically use cream in this, but not for the 30-Day)

ESSENTIAL OILS – RECIPES AND MIXTURES

Fresh Start Bath Soak

(enough for 2 soaks)

1 cup Epsom salt

1 cup dead sea salt

½ cup baking soda

10 drops Eucalyptus essential oil

10 drops Lavender essential oil

½ ounce peppermint leaves

Mix Epsom salt, dead sea salt, and baking soda in large bowl. Stir in peppermint leaves and essential oils thoroughly.

Store in glass air tight container.

** This is a detox soak – so drink plenty of water after a 30-minute soak.**

Bug/Mosquito Spray

½ cup distilled water

5 drops each of the following essential oils:

- Purification
- Lemongrass
- Palo Santo
- Citronella

Pain Relief

1 cup coconut oil

10 drops each of the following essential oils:

- Valor
- PanAway
- Peppermint
- Copaiba
- Lemongrass

Sleep

½ cup coconut oil

15 drops of Cedarwood oil

15 drops of Lavender oil

15 drops of Peace & Calming oil

Rosemary Lemon Cashews

10 oz raw cashews

2 Tbsp extra virgin olive oil

3 sprigs fresh rosemary (leaves removed)

Peel of 1 lemon (zest)

4 drops Rosemary oil

2 drops Lemon oil

¾ tsp coarse sea salt

- Preheat oven to 375°
- Place nuts on baking sheet and roast for 8-10 minutes.
- While nuts are roasting, warm olive oil, fresh rosemary, and lemon zest in skillet over medium heat until sizzling and fragrant. Add cashews.
- Remove from heat. Stir in oils and salt. Enjoy!

HEALING FOOD SHOPPING LIST

VEGETABLES

- ☐ Artichoke
- ☐ Arugula
- ☐ Asparagus
- ☐ Avocados
- ☐ Beets / Beet Greens
- ☐ Bell Peppers
- ☐ Bok Choy
- ☐ Broccoli
- ☐ Broccoli Rabe
- ☐ Brussels Sprouts
- ☐ Cabbage
- ☐ Carrots
- ☐ Celery
- ☐ Collard Greens
- ☐ Cucumbers
- ☐ Eggplant
- ☐ Garlic
- ☐ Green Beans
- ☐ Jerusalem Artichoke
- ☐ Kale
- ☐ Mushrooms
- ☐ Olives
- ☐ Onions
- ☐ Parsnip
- ☐ Peppers (all kinds)
- ☐ Pumpkin
- ☐ Radish
- ☐ Romaine Lettuce
- ☐ Sea Vegetables
- ☐ Spinach
- ☐ Squash
- ☐ Tomatoes
- ☐ Turnip Greens
- ☐ Watercress
- ☐ Wheat Grass

In Moderation:

- ☐ Brown / Wild Rice
- ☐ Beans
- ☐ Sweet Potatoes
- ☐ Quinoa

FISH (Wild Caught only, NO Farm Raised)

- ☐ Anchovies
- ☐ Bass
- ☐ Cod
- ☐ Grouper
- ☐ Haddock
- ☐ Halibut
- ☐ Herring
- ☐ Mackerel
- ☐ Mahi Mahi
- ☐ Red Snapper
- ☐ Salmon
- ☐ Sardines
- ☐ Seabass
- ☐ Trout
- ☐ Tuna
- ☐ Walleye
- ✘ NO Shellfish

DAIRY (Raw, or Low-Temp Processed)

- ☐ A2 Cows Milk
- ☐ A2 Cows Cheese
- ☐ A2 Cows Amasai
- ☐ Goats Milk
- ☐ Goats Cheese
- ☐ Kefir (Cultured Goat Milk)
- ☐ Sheep Cheese
- ☐ Sheep Yogurt
- ☐ Any Other Raw Dairy

MEAT (Organic, Grassfed)

- ☐ Beef
- ☐ Bison
- ☐ Chicken
- ☐ Duck
- ☐ Eggs
- ☐ Lamb
- ☐ Quail and other wild game
- ☐ Turkey
- ☐ Venison and other wild game
- ✘ NO Pork

NUTS AND SEEDS

- ☐ Almonds
- ☐ Brazil Nuts
- ☐ Chia Seeds
- ☐ Flax Seeds
- ☐ Hemp Seeds
- ☐ Hazelnuts
- ☐ Macadamia Nuts
- ☐ Pecans
- ☐ Pine Nuts
- ☐ Pistachios
- ☐ Pumpkin Seeds
- ☐ Sesame Seeds
- ☐ Walnuts
- ☐ Nut Butters
- ☐ Seed Butters
- ✘ NO Peanuts

FATS / OILS (Organic, Unrefined)

- ☐ Avocado Oil
- ☐ Almond Oil
- ☐ Butter (pastured)
- ☐ Coconut Butter
- ☐ Coconut Oil / Milk
- ☐ Ghee
- ☐ Grapeseed Oil
- ☐ Macadamia Oil
- ☐ Olive Oil
- ☐ Palm Oil
- ☐ Sesame Oil
- ☐ Walnut Oil
- ✘ NO Canola Oil

FRUITS (Preferred)

- ☐ Blackberries
- ☐ Blueberries
- ☐ Cranberries
- ☐ Goji Berries
- ☐ Raspberries
- ☐ Strawberries

In Moderation:

- ☐ African Mango
- ☐ Apple
- ☐ Apricot
- ☐ Banana
- ☐ Cantaloupe
- ☐ Camu-Camu
- ☐ Cherries
- ☐ Coconuts
- ☐ Figs
- ☐ Grapefruit
- ☐ Grapes
- ☐ Indian Gooseberry
- ☐ Lemon
- ☐ Lime
- ☐ Mango
- ☐ Nectarine
- ☐ Orange
- ☐ Papaya
- ☐ Peaches
- ☐ Pears
- ☐ Pineapple
- ☐ Plums
- ☐ Pomegranate
- ☐ Rhubarb
- ☐ Watermelon
  - All other fruits

OCCASIONAL INDULGENCES

- ☐ Dark Chocolate (60-80% or more cacao)
- ✗ NO Milk Chocolate

SPICES AND HERBS

- ☐ Basil
- ☐ Black Pepper
- ☐ Cayenne Pepper
- ☐ Chili Pepper
- ☐ Cilantro
- ☐ Coriander Seeds
- ☐ Cinnamon
- ☐ Cloves
- ☐ Cumin
- ☐ Dill
- ☐ Fennel
- ☐ Garlic
- ☐ Ginger
- ☐ Mint
- ☐ Mustard seeds
- ☐ Nutmeg
- ☐ Oregano
- ☐ Paprika
- ☐ Parsley
- ☐ Peppermint
- ☐ Rosemary
- ☐ Sage
- ☐ Tarragon
- ☐ Thyme
- ☐ Turmeric

CONDIMENTS

- ☐ Apple Cider Vinegar
- ☐ Balsamic Vinegar
- ☐ Coconut Vinegar
- ☐ Coconut Aminos
- ☐ Cocoa
- ☐ Extracts (Vanilla / Almond)
- ☐ Guacamole
- ☐ Hummus
- ☐ Mustard (Stone Ground)
- ☐ Mayo (Grapeseed Oil)
- ☐ Salsa
- ☐ Sea Salt
- ☐ Tamari

BEVERAGES

- ☐ Almond Milk
- ☐ Cashew Milk
- ☐ Coconut Kefir
- ☐ Coconut Milk
- ☐ Cultured Whey
- ☐ Hemp Milk
- ☐ Herbal Teas
- ☐ Kombucha
- ☐ Raw Vegetable Juices
- ☐ Sparkling Water
- ☐ Spring Water (or Filtered)

SWEETENERS

In Moderation

- ☐ Figs
- ☐ Maple Syrup (pure, organic)
- ☐ Medjool Dates
- ☐ Monk Fruit
- ☐ Raw Honey
- ☐ Stevia

SUPPLEMENTS

- ☐ Brown Rice Protein Powder
- ☐ Digestive Enzymes
- ☐ Greens Powder
- ☐ Omega-3 Fish Oil or Flaxseed Oil
- ☐ Pea Protein Powder
- ☐ Plant-Based Protein
- ☐ Probiotics
- ☐ Vitamin D-3
- ☐ Whey Protein Concentrate Powder (Grassfed)
- ☐ Whole Food-Based Multi-Vitamin

Edited version of Dr. Axe's Healing Food Shopping List

Glycemic Index
CardioProtective Lifestyle Program

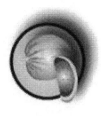

The Glycemic Index (GI) is a measure of how much your blood sugar level rises after a food is ingested. High GI foods cause blood sugar to rise quickly, whereas a food with a low GI causes a smaller rise in blood sugar and may help control established diabetes, aid in weight loss, and lower cholesterol.

Grain/Starch
LOW
- Rice bran 27
- Barley, pearled 36
- Spaghetti, protein enriched 38
- Fettuccine 46
- Spaghetti, wholemeal 53
- Fruit 'n Oats 55
- Spaghetti, white 59
- Wheat kernels 59
- All-Bran 60
- Macaroni 64
- Linguine 65
- Rye Kernel bread 65
- Instant noodles 67
- Oat bran bread 68
- Bulgur 68
- Mixed grain bread 69
- Pumpernickel bread 77
- Bran Buds 77
- Special K 78
- Oat Bran 78
- Popcorn 79
- Rice, brown 79
- Muesli 80

MODERATE
- Pita bread, white 82
- Bran Chex 83
- Rice, white 83
- Cornflakes 87
- Hamburger bun 87
- Oatmeal 87
- Rye flour bread 92

Grain/Starch (cont.)
MODERATE (cont.)
- Oat kernel bread 93
- Kellogg's Couscous 93
- High Fibre Rye Crisp 93
- Nutri-grain 94
- Life 94

HIGH
- Barley flour bread 95
- Gnocchi 95
- Grapenuts 96
- Stoned Wheat Thins 96
- Wheat bread 97
- Taco shells 97
- Shredded Wheat 98
- Cream of Wheat 99
- White bread 100
- Golden Grahams 102
- Water Crackers 102
- Bagel, white 103
- Kaiser roll 104
- Bread stuffing 106
- Cheerios 106
- Total 109
- Breakfast bar 109
- Rice Cakes 110
- Post Flakes 114
- Rice Krispies 117
- Cornflakes 119
- Rice Chex 127
- Rice, instant 128
- French baguette 136

Vegetable
LOW
- Peas, dried 32
- Tomato soup 54
- Marrowfat, dried 56
- Peas, green 68
- Carrots 70
- Yam 77
- Sweet potato 77
- Sweet Corn 78
- Potato, white, boiled 81
- Potato, new 81

MODERATE
- Beets 91
- Potato, canned 97

HIGH
- Potato, mashed 100
- Rutabaga 103
- Pumpkin 107
- French fries 107
- Potato, microwaved 117
- Potato, instant 116
- Potato, baked 121
- Parsnips 139

Fruit
LOW
- Cherries 32
- Grapefruit 36
- Apricots, dried 44
- Pear, fresh 53
- Apple 54
- Plum 55
- Peach, fresh 60
- Orange 63
- Grapes 66
- Peach, canned 67
- Kiwifruit 75
- Banana 77

MODERATE
- Fruit cocktail 79
- Mango 80
- Apricots, fresh 82
- Cantaloupe 91
- Raisins 91
- Pineapple 94

HIGH
- Watermelon 103
- Dates 141

Dairy
LOW
- Yogurt, low fat, sweetened 20
- Milk, chocolate, artificially sweetened 34
- Milk, regular 39
- Soy milk 43
- Milk, skim/nonfat 46
- Yogurt, low fat, fruit sugar sweet 47
- Milk, chocolate, sugar sweetened 49

MODERATE
- Ice cream, low fat 71

HIGH
- Ice cream 87

Protein
LOW
- Peanuts 21
- Beans, dried, not specified 40
- Lentils, not specified 41
- Kidney beans 41
- Butter beans 43
- Split peas, yellow, boiled 45
- Lima beans, baby, frozen 46
- Chick peas (garbanzo beans) 47
- Navy beans 54
- Pinto beans 55
- Black-eyed beans 59
- Chick peas, canned 60
- Lentil soup, canned 63
- Pinto beans, canned 64
- Baked beans 69
- Kidney beans, canned 74
- Lentils, canned 74

MODERATE
- Split pea soup 86
- Black bean soup 92
- Green pea soup, canned 94

Sweets
LOW
- Fructose 31
- Strawberry jam 51
- Cake, sponge 66
- Ice cream, low fat 71
- Cake, pound 77
- Oatmeal cookies 79

MODERATE
- High Fructose Power Bar 81
- Pastry 84
- Muesli Bars 84
- Ice cream 87
- Muffins 88
- Sucrose (table sugar) 89
- Corn Syrup 90
- Shortbread 91

HIGH
- Cake, angel food 95
- Croissant 96
- Corn chips 105
- Graham Wafers 106
- Donut 108
- Waffles 109
- Vanilla Wafers 110
- Tapioca boiled with milk 115
- Pretzels 116
- Honey 126
- Glucose 138
- Maltose 152
- Tofu frozen dessert, non-dairy 164

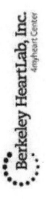

Berkeley HeartLab, Inc.
4myheart Center

GLYCEMIC INDEX

Feeling Words

Mad	Sad	Glad	Afraid	Confused	Ashamed	Lonely
A Little	*A Little*	*A Little*	*A Little*	*A Little*	*A Little*	*A Little*
Bothered	Down	At ease	Uneasy	Curious	Uncomfortable	Out-of-place
Ruffled	Blue	Secure	Apprehensive	Uncertain	Awkward	Left-out
Irritate	Somber	Comfortable	Careful	Ambivalent	Clumsy	Unheeded
Displeased	Low	Relaxed	Cautious	Doubtful	Self-conscious	Lonesome
Annoyed	Glum	Contented	Hesitant	Unsettled	Disconcerted	Distant
Steamed	Lonely	Optimistic	Tense	Hesitant	Chagrined	Remote
Irked	Disappointed	Satisfied	Anxious	Perplexed	Abashed	Invisible
Perturbed	Worn-out	Refreshed	Nervous	Puzzled	Embarrassed	Unimportant
Frustrated	Melancholy	Stimulated	Edgy	Muddled	Flustered	Cut-off
Angry	Downhearted	Pleased	Distressed	Distracted	Sorry	Excluded
Fed-up	Unhappy	Warm	Scared	Flustered	Apologetic	Insignificant
Disgusted	Dissatisfied	Snug	Frightened	Jumbled	Ashamed	Ignored
Indignant	Gloomy	Happy	Repulsed	Unfocused	Regretful	Neglected
Ticked-off	Mournful	Encouraged	Agitated	Fragmented	Remorseful	Separated
Bristling	Grieved	Tickled	Afraid	Dismayed	Guilty	Removed
Fuming	Depressed	Proud	Shocked	Insecure	Disgusted	Dislocated
Explosive	Lousy	Cheerful	Alarmed	Dazed	Belittled	Isolated
Enraged	Crushed	Thrilled	Overwhelmed	Bewildered	Humiliated	Rejected
Irate	Defeated	Delighted	Frantic	Lost	Violated	Unwanted
Incensed	Dejected	Joyful	Panic-stricken	Stunned	Dirty	Deserted
Burned	Empty	Elated	Horrified	Chaotic	Mortified	Outcast
Burned-up	Wretched	Exhilarated	Petrified	Torn	Defiled	Abandoned
Outraged	Despairing	Overjoyed	Terrified	Baffled	Devastated	Desolate
Furious	Devastated	Ecstatic	Numb	Dumbfounded	Degraded	Forsaken
A Lot	*A Lot*	*A Lot*	*A Lot*	*A Lot*	*A Lot*	*A Lot*

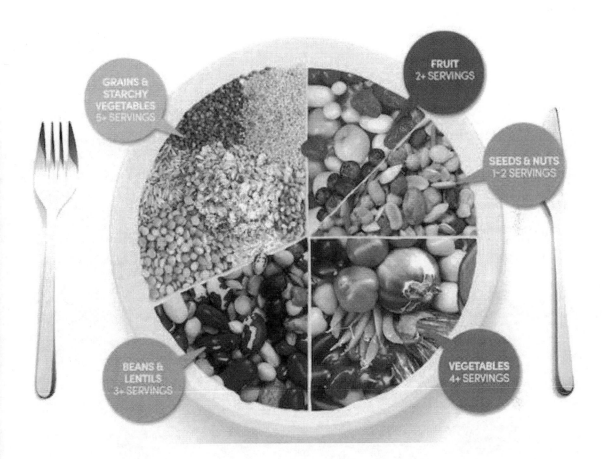

GRAINS &
STARCHY
VEGETABLES
5+ SERVINGS

FRUIT
2+ SERVINGS

SEEDS & NUTS
1–2 SERVINGS

BEANS &
LENTILS
3+ SERVINGS

VEGETABLES
4+ SERVINGS

VEGAN PROTEINS
EQUIVALENT TO 1 OZ. OF MEAT

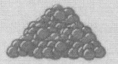

1/2 Cup Cooked Quinoa

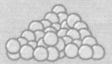

3/4 cup Cooked Lentils

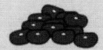

1/4 Cup Cooked Black Beans

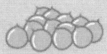

1/4 Cup Cooked Chickpeas OR 1/2 Cup Hummus

4 Tablespoons Chia

1 1/2 Tablespoons Hemp Seeds

1oz (or 1/4 Cup) Raw Almonds or 1 TBSP Almond Butter

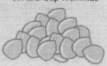

1 1/2 Oz Pumpkin Seeds

5 Tablespoons of Sesame, Sunflower, or Poppy Seeds

1 1/4 Cup Brown Rice

Leafy Greens: 5 Cups Chopped Kale or 1/4 Cup Chopped Spinach

1 Tablespoon Powdered Spirulina

HOW MUCH PROTEIN DO VEGANS NEED?

FOR HEALTHY ADULTS: BODY WEIGHT x 0.8g= DAILY PROTEIN TARGET
(TO GAIN MUSCLE: 70-120g protein/daily)

This means that if you weigh 175 pounds, you'll need approx. 64g of protein a day. If 64g sounds like a lot of protein to obtain in a day, try this menu to get started.

THIS IS WHAT A PERFECT DAY OF VEGAN PROTEIN LOOKS LIKE

BREAKFAST
APPROX. 15 G PROTEIN

Blueberry Fuel Smoothie
1 cup frozen blueberries
1 cup vanilla almond milk
5 cups raw spinach

Blend together until smooth.

SNACK: APPROX. 7 GRAMS PROTEIN
2 Tbsp Almond Butter & Apples

LUNCH APPROX. 17 GRAMS PROTEIN

Chickpea Quinoa Tabbouleh
1/2 cup cooked chickpeas
½ cup cooked quinoa
¼ cup parsley, chopped
Juice and zest of 1 lemon
2 tablespoons olive oil
1 tomato, diced

Toss together.
Salt and pepper to taste.

DINNER APPROX. 25 GRAMS PROTEIN

Sunny Rice Bowl
2 tablespoons coconut oil
¼ onion, finely diced
1 clove garlic, finely chopped
4 cups chopped kale
1 cup lentils, cooked
1 cup brown rice, cooked
1 tablespoons hemp seeds

Heat coconut oil in a large skillet. Add diced onion, garlic, and kale. Saute until tender. Add lentils. Serve over brown rice. Sprinkle with hemp seeds. Salt and pepper to taste.

TOTAL PROTEIN INTAKE: APPROX. 64 GRAMS PROTEIN

Yurielkaim.com

USEFUL INFORMATION ON NUTS

ALMONDS

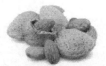

Good Source Of:
Calcium, iron, fiber, vitamin E, riboflavin, magnesium, phosphorus, manganese

FAT: 14g
PROTEIN: 6g
FIBER: 3.5g

163 Calories

CASHEWS

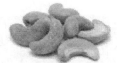

Good Source Of:
Magnesium, phosphorus, copper, iron

FAT: 13g
PROTEIN: 4.5g
FIBER: 1g

163 Calories

HAZELNUTS

Good Source Of:
Magnesium, copper, manganese, phosphorus, vitamin E, selenium, fiber

FAT: 17g
PROTEIN: 4g
FIBER: 2.5g

178 Calories

MACADAMIA NUTS

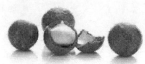

Good Source Of:
Magnesium, thiamin, potassium, manganese

FAT: 22g
PROTEIN: 2g
FIBER: 2g

204 Calories

PEANUTS

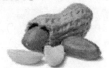

Good Source Of:
Protein, niacin, vitamin E, folate, magnesium, phosphorus, manganese, copper

FAT: 14g
PROTEIN: 6.5g
FIBER: 2.5g

166 Calories

PECANS

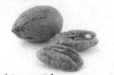

Good Source Of:
Fiber, magnesium, phosphorus, copper, zinc, manganese

FAT: 21g
PROTEIN: 3g
FIBER: 3g

199 Calories

PINE NUTS

Good Source Of:
Vitamin E, vitamin K, magnesium, phosphorus, potassium, zinc, copper

FAT: 19g
PROTEIN: 4g
FIBER: 1g

188 Calories

PISTACHIOS

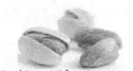

Good Source Of:
Fiber, thiamin, vitamin B6, phosphorus, copper, manganese

FAT: 13g
PROTEIN: 6g
FIBER: 3g

161 Calories

WALNUTS

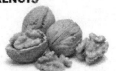

Good Source Of:
Protein, vitamin B6, magnesium, phosphorus, copper, manganese, selenium

FAT: 17g
PROTEIN: 7g
FIBER: 2g

173 Calories

Serving Size: 30 g

For recipes, health advice and food inspiration visit
http://adrianlupsa.wordpress.com

211

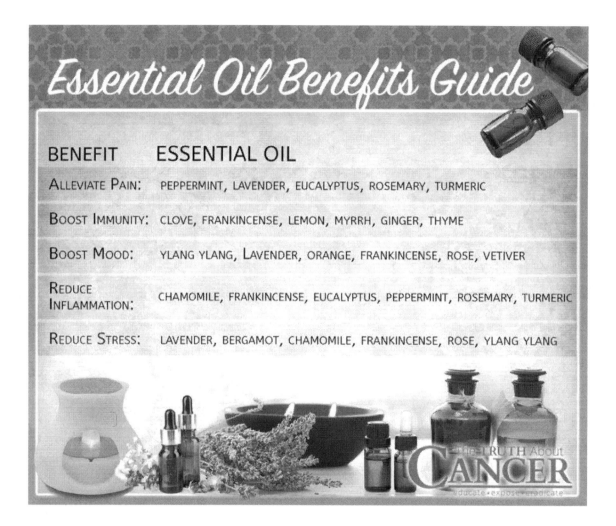

Essential Oil Benefits Guide

BENEFIT	ESSENTIAL OIL
ALLEVIATE PAIN:	PEPPERMINT, LAVENDER, EUCALYPTUS, ROSEMARY, TURMERIC
BOOST IMMUNITY:	CLOVE, FRANKINCENSE, LEMON, MYRRH, GINGER, THYME
BOOST MOOD:	YLANG YLANG, LAVENDER, ORANGE, FRANKINCENSE, ROSE, VETIVER
REDUCE INFLAMMATION:	CHAMOMILE, FRANKINCENSE, EUCALYPTUS, PEPPERMINT, ROSEMARY, TURMERIC
REDUCE STRESS:	LAVENDER, BERGAMOT, CHAMOMILE, FRANKINCENSE, ROSE, YLANG YLANG

The TRUTH About CANCER
educate • expose • eradicate

MEET THE AUTHORS

LILLIAN M. EASTERLY-SMITH'S experience spans over 30 years. She is the Founder and Director of LifeCare Christian Center – a care center in the Metro-Detroit area that takes a whole-person approach to helping people: body, soul and spirit. She has served as speaker, teacher and leader of pilot programs, ministries and groups for those dealing with various forms of abuse, addictions and dysfunctional family issues, as well as counseling individuals and couples one-on-one. Lillian leads groups, leads worship, organizes retreats, trains leaders and teaches in many workshops, seminars and classes that offer information, support and help for lifestyle changes that last.

Lillian has volunteered/been employed at four major area churches where she developed care ministries that included a vibrant lay counseling ministry as well as programs for spiritual formation and discipleship. Lillian has managed staff and volunteer teams of over 300. She has a degree in Counseling/Psychology and Biblical Studies, is a Board Certified Pastoral Counselor, licensed Pastor & Chaplain, a Certified Health & Wellness Coach as well as a Fitness/Exercise Instructor. She is a much sought-after speaker for seminars, workshops and retreats. She has published two books prior to this current release and has served and currently serves in three Board of Director positions for non-profit organizations. Lillian is also a member of two area Health Coalitions for city-wide efforts in making communities healthy in Westland and Canton/Plymouth, Michigan.

Lillian believes in living life to the fullest. Her desire is to see Christ-followers live a life of purpose and adventure that comes from a place of health and wholeness. Lillian and Mike continue to pursue all that God has for them in ministry and at the same time enjoy life, each other, friends and family. Their hope and prayer are that the things they love: God (#1), the Word, music, books, learning and giving would influence others to live a life fully surrendered to God's plan.

213

Life Verse: The pulse of Lillian's heart stems from one of her life verses found in Romans 8:28 (NIV) "And we know that in all things God works for the good of those who love him, who have been called according to his purpose."

MICHAEL D. SMITH, LIFE COACH, AND HEALTH & WELLNESS COACH – Mike Smith has been coaching adolescents and adults for over 9 years. His training comes through CTI (Coaches Training Institute) as well as Light University's Life Coaching and Health & Wellness Coaching Programs.

As a life coach, teacher, speaker and group leader for LifeCare Christian Center, Mike has had the privilege of witnessing the healing power and love of Jesus Christ in the lives of individuals locally as well as internationally. Mike has had the opportunity to minister in Gambia, Ghana and multiple regions within the United States. He says, "whether around the block or around the globe, God calls us to use the gifts He's given us for the benefit of those in need, and most importantly, to expand His kingdom.

Mike is a former Team Beach Body Coach, Life Enrichment Director for a senior independent living facility where he taught exercise/health & wellness classes along with writing the life enrichment column in their monthly newsletter. He was a ghost writer for a publication authored by a world renowned fitness trainer and motivational speaker and currently serves in two Board of Director positions for non-profit organizations.

Mike's love for animals, children (especially those in orphanages), different cultures, the outdoors and being active – whether it be tending to animals at an area farm, running, biking or competing in obstacle course events – keeps his desire for variety fueled. He also loves the arts (drama team participation in several churches was an outlet) and is a musician who has been playing guitar and drumming (of which Lillian is his biggest fan) all his life in bands, churches, LifeCare and other venues.

Mike believes the world needs "up reach" more than outreach. Our hands only give what is temporary, but what the hand of God gives is eternal. He is passionate about Christian apologetics, (evidence-based knowledge of the Christian faith) and loves teaching and sharing it with others.

Life Verse: The pulse of Mike's heart stems from one of his life verses found in Galatians 2:20b (NIV) "…The life I now live in the body, I live by faith in the Son of God, who loved me and gave himself for me."

The blessing of his life is to be able to do God's work hand-in-hand and heart-to-heart with his wife, Lillian.

ACKNOWLEDGMENTS

As we considered the countless family, friends, and ministry partners who have poured time, talent, treasure, and prayer into our lives over the years, we came to the very humble conclusion that it would take 100 pages to include each and every one. All of you are an undeserved blessing and vital part of our journey in life. We are so thankful for such favor from God. It is only by His provision and grace that we have those of you in our lives as well as the abilities and knowledge He has given to complete this endeavor.

We would, however, like to thank those who have been directly involved in the making of this book as well as the couple that inspired us at the beginning.

Kelly Hawkins – Our editor, mistake detective, and detail master. As big picture thinkers, we are forever grateful for your attention to detail, your creative mind, and your relentless efforts to make this book worthy of print. Your life exemplifies doing all things for the glory of God.

Chuck and Sheila Herr – It is one thing to teach, and another to practice. In doing both, your wisdom, heart, and action in sharing the truth about honoring God with our bodies gave us the kick start that we needed 10-11 years ago to put our wellness journey into 2nd, 3rd, and 4th gear.

Our deepest and greatest thanks, gratitude, and praise belong only to Jesus, our Savior, who willingly gave His life as a ransom for us. In every breath, every task, and all the gifts we possess, we desire to give Him the glory. We will boast only in the cross of Christ. He is the vine, we are the branches, and without Him, we can do nothing.

RESOURCES

Just a few people and organizations we follow as well as places you can get additional support and information:

DR. MERCOLA	DR. JOCKERS
DR. AXE	DR. BROWNSTEIN
FOOD BABE	JORDAN RUBIN
DR. REX RUSSELL	DR. DON CULBERT
TAMARA ST. JOHN	DR. J FUHRMAN
MIKE ADAMS – THE HEALTH RANGER	DR. T COLIN CAMPBELL
TY BOLLINGER – THE TRUTH ABOUT CANCER	FORKS OVER KNIVES
DR. BEN LERNER – MAXIMIZED LIVING	HALLELUJAH ACRES
DR. CYNTHIA SHAFT	DR. CHRIS NIEDZINSKI

We are not in 100% agreement with any of the above methods, philosophies, and especially spiritual positions of these authors, doctors, teachers, and ministries, but they have been helpful in discovering truth that helps us continue our research and application of truth in our own lives that can be supported by science.

OUR FACEBOOK PAGE: LIFECARE – LIVING WELL: HEALTH & WELLNESS GROUP

OTHER OPTIONS:

- 30-Day JUMPSTART YOUR JOURNEY – LIFESTYLE CHANGE (the majority of the program is in this book)
- INDIVIDUALIZED PERSONAL HEALTH & WELLNESS COACHING (includes a nutrition assessment and personalized program) – by phone, email, face time, Skype, Facebook (contact us via email for more info: Info.LifeCareCC@gmail.com)

- BABY STEP PROGRAM (included in this book)
- ONLINE PRIVATE FACEBOOK CLASS – VIDEO INSTRUCTION, slides, handouts, recipes, nutritional assessment, and more!
- FIT 'n' FAITH Retreats – 2x's per year (CHECK OUR WEBSITE FOR DATES under Living Well Programs) http://lifecarechristiancenter.org/living_well.aspx

REFERENCES

American Heart Association. http://sugarscience.ucsf.edu/the-growing-concern-of-overconsumption/#.Wqhu2kxFzIU.

Axe/Rubin/eating window. https://draxe.com/time-restricted-eating/. https://www.facebook.com/JordanRubinOfficial.

Benard, Solomon. http://ezinearticles.com/?Timeless-Lessons-From-the-7-Principles-of-the-Eagle&id=2639477.

Better Nutrition. https://www.betternutrition.com/ask-the-naturopath/preventing-cancer.

Brownstein, Dr. David. https://w3.brownsteinhealth.com/Health/DRB/Offers/DRB-Leaky-Gut-Trial?dkt_nbr=030603ovejvt&msclkid=2dd55ce295cf1e838b100620d16bfd14.

Campbell, T. Colin, PhD. http://extension.oregonstate.edu/coos/sites/default/files/FFE/documents/animal_vs_plant_protein._t_colin_campbell.pdf.

CDC/obesity. https://www.cdc.gov/obesity/data/adult.html. https://www.cdc.gov/diabetes/pubs/pdf/ndfs_2011.pdf.

Cloud, Henry. https://www.goodreads.com/author/quotes/1114699.Henry_Cloud?page=3.

Clum, Dr. Don. https://www.facebook.com/don.clum.10. https://www.facebook.com/don.clum/. https://www.facebook.com/search/top/?q=%20don%20clum%20fasting.

Doctorshealth/B17. https://www.doctorshealthpress.com/food-and-nutrition-articles/vitamin-b17-laetrile-foods/.

Dr. Axe's Healing Food Shopping List. http://draxe.s3.amazonaws.com/Ebooks/Dr.%20Axe%20-%20Healing%20Food%20Shopping%20List.pdf .

Eldredge, John. http://www.notable-quotes.com/e/eldredge_john.html.

Fitlife/superfoods. http://fitlife.tv/superfoods-that-are-actually-healthier-than-kale_original/nutrition/.

Food Babe/sugar. https://foodbabe.com/how-to-beat-sugar-cravings-addiction-for-good/.

Franklin, Benjamin. https://www.brainyquote.com/quotes/benjamin_franklin_140816.

Hallelujah/depression. http://www.myhdiet.com/healthnews/health-news/truth-about-depression-natural-solution/.

Healthy Eating. http://healthyeating.sfgate.com/roles-protein-play-body-3918.html.

Hyatt, Michael. https://beyondthetodolist.com/focus-michael-hyatt-on-energy-clarity-and-focus-bttdl191/. Phrase also attributed to Tony Schwartz. http://engageforsuccess.org/wp-content/uploads/2015/12/Manage_Your_Energy_Not_Your_Time_HBR.pdf.

Hyman, Dr. Mark/sugar. http://drhyman.com/blog/2014/12/18/7-ways-reverse-obesity-diabetes/.

Institute of Medicine. https://www.nap.edu/read/10490/chapter/32?term=protein+#1324.

Jockers/sugar. https://drjockers.com/destructive-sugar-impact/.

King, Dr. Martin Luther, Jr. https://www.youtube.com/watch?time_continue=128&v=MFOFs0iAwDg.

Maxwell, John. http://hereiamlord7.blogspot.com/2007/09/.

Mercola/B17. https://articles.mercola.com/sites/articles/archive/2014/10/18/laetrile-cancer-research-cover-up.aspx.

Mercola/balsamic. https://recipes.mercola.com/balsamic-drizzled-Brussels-sprouts-recipe.aspx.

Mercola/sugar. https://articles.mercola.com/sites/articles/archive/2016/09/07/recommended-sugar-intake.aspx.

Myhdiet/protein. Entire protein section through this reference is taken from http://www.myhdiet.com/healthnews/ampm/how-much-protein-do-you-really-need-every-day/.

New Scientist. https://www.newscientist.com/article/dn16397-top-11-compounds-in-us-drinking-water.

One Green Planet. Entire protein section following Myhdiet/protein section through this reference is taken from https://www.onegreenplanet.org/vegan-food/how-to-tell-if-youre-getting-enough-protein/comment-page-5/.

Ramsey, Dave. https://www.daveramsey.com/blog/hurdles-to-financial-peace/.

Sears. https://www.askdrsears.com/topics/feeding-eating/family-nutrition/sugar/harmful-effects-excess-sugar.

"Several Years Ago I Read a Story." God Always Has a Plan B, by Luci Swindoll, Zondervan Publishing House, 1999, p.27.

TTAC/emotions. https://thetruthaboutcancer.com/emotional-clearing/.

TTAC/detox. https://thetruthaboutcancer.com/natural-body-detox/.

Wikipedia/Complete Protein. https://en.wikipedia.org/wiki/Complete_protein.

Wirthlin, Joseph B. https://www.brainyquote.com/quotes/joseph_b_wirthlin_645972.

Wolfe/avocado. https://www.davidwolfe.com/avocado-seeds-health-benefits/.

Wolfe/superfoods. https://www.davidwolfe.com/superfoods-best-bites-for-buck/.

Wooden, John. Quote. https://www.goodreads.com/quotes/63067-it-s-what-you-learn-after-you-know-it-all-that.

Wright, Steven. http://www.weather.net/zarg/ZarPages/stevenWright.html.

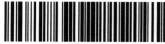

Made in the USA
Columbia, SC
27 May 2018